HOW TO FEMINIZE

YOUR BODY:

A helpful guide for Crossdressers
By
Martine M Song

Disclaimer

The following text contains various suggestions and techniques for feminizing your body. The author is not a trained counsellor or therapist for transgender issues or medically qualified. If you are seeking permanent transition or hormone treatments or surgery of any kind, please consult with a qualified practitioner. Padding, tucking, taping, or waist training techniques are conducted at your own risk. The author accepts no responsibility or liability whatsoever for your dressing activities.

CONTENTS

Part I
Introduction

What are girls made of?
Sugar and Spice and all things nice.
That's what girls are made of

[Old rhyme]

Chapter 1 Introduction

Hi and welcome. You probably guessed from the title that this is a book about how to enjoy your feminine feelings and bring out your inner womanliness. In short, the topic is male-to-female transformation. Some people call it makeover, that works too. The text is written predominantly from the view that you are new to crossdressing and feminization but want to develop a female persona of some kind be it permanent or just for a temporary indulgence. It can also be used by supporters, helpers, or indeed mistresses as a kind of manual or workbook to help socialise you into feminine ways. If you are an old hand then you may also find a few helpful tips or insights that will further enhance your look, style, or dressing technique.

There can be a whole bunch of reasons why you might be interested in feminizing yourself so let's be clear at the outset. This is a how to book. We don't spend a lot of time on psychology, whys, or what-ifs. We don't do any handwringing or worry about what got you here. Not that these aren't important topics it is just that there are better resources available.

You are who you are. Our starting point is simply to accept that your feminine feelings are real. That they well up every now and then, if not constantly, and need some outlet for you to feel congruent with yourself. If you feel a little happier as a result of reading this book and putting bits of it into action that's great.

The four pillars of feminization

The four pillars hold the key to successful feminization. Each stage of development lays a foundation to get the best look you can. The foundations include body shape and deportment or how you move; face makeup and hair styling; clothing, stockings, and heels; and voice or how you sound.

You wouldn't think about choosing clothes if you didn't know your body type and you wouldn't rush into makeup without applying proper foundation and concealer first. Likewise, you wouldn't dress without due regard to the right undergarment such as the type of bra or panties to avoid unsightly straps or lines. Similarly, you'd be careful of how you moved and held yourself depending on whether your outfit was revealing or demure, or if you were wearing flats or heels. And, of course once you have perfected your look you don't want to let it all be for nothing by sounding like a nightclub bouncer.

Rather than cramming all these topics into one volume we want to give them the detail they deserve. This is often the problem with books on crossdressing. They cover everything in brief leaving you lots to discover on your own. And, as we all know there can be a huge difference between the vision you have in your head and what turns out to be reality. Our goal is to connect the two. And for that you need options and details.

This book covers two of the essential pillars of feminization. Our focus is how you can get a pleasing feminine shape. In other words, boobs, butts, body, and other bits. We also look a little at fashion, underwear and that important topic of walking in heels. The other two pillars: Makeup and hair styling and feminizing your voice are not covered in this volume. These are huge and important topics which I hope to cover in sister volumes.

Femininity

Femininity is a set of attributes that we normally associate with girls or women. These attributes include certain behaviours, roles, and expectations. Femininity also includes appearance and qualities such as delicacy, softness and prettiness.

Physically this involves attention to hair style and length, a lack of body and facial hair, body shape, hygiene and neatness. Fashion wise it extends to the choice of certain colours, makeup, clothes, perfumes and accessories. Posture and how you move are also important factors. All these things together contribute to recognising someone as not just female but also feminine. These characteristics of femininity give us a shopping list for the things we will need, and the changes required to get the best outcome of your makeover.

Who is this book for?

There are several categories of people that will benefit from the information contained in these pages. Leaving aside the merely curious we can divide them into three main types.

Transvestites – this is an older term for the more politically correct phrase crossdresser. We keep it only to make a distinction. Though most crossdressers derive some pleasure from dressing in female clothes what we want to capture here is the group that dresses mainly for sexual excitement or arousal. In general, fetishes are not problematic unless a person experiences distress resulting from the desire. This book doesn't focus on erotic activities per se but it will help you be more authentic when you play and we'll give you some hints as to how dressing can be used to enhance your desires. If we help you feel sexier and more sensual that is a result.

Crossdressers– is the more modern term for wearing clothes of the opposite sex. In this group we include people that just like to dress for social reasons or to explore their feminine side. The key here is the outside presentation of your female persona. When the chief reason for dressing is not erotic then crossdressing is not a fetish. Crossdressing can of course be a first step in a more permanent transition, but it doesn't have to be. Many people are happy as Tgirls, Shemales, Ladyboys (or more colourfully chicks with dicks). Our objective is to give you a range of options to perfect your look.

Transgenders-include people that are following a transition, taking hormones, and are on a path to body modification so they can live happily as female. You may feel that nature gave you the wrong body (gender dysphoria). That's a complex psychological issue where distress is caused by the difference between your sex assigned at birth and your experienced or expressed gender. We don't discuss that in detail here. But hopefully this book will help your socialisation as female. You'll need to decide which bits to skip and which to retain depending on the stage of your transition. Generally, as your path develops, you'll need less and less on looking physically female but more on how to dress and act to bring out your femininity in other ways.

Another group of possible readers are biological females or genetic girls (gee-gees) that struggle with femininity. Usually this is because you missed out on some of the socialisation when growing up. Maybe your mother wasn't that girly, you lived in a more masculine environment, or just dismissed girl stuff as a bit fluffy. Maybe you want to find a partner and think that looking and behaving more feminine will work for you. That's okay too. Hopefully there will be something here to help. There are lots of tips, tricks, and advice to realise your ambitions in the pages that follow. Use what you need and forget the rest.

This list is not exhaustive. You might be a mixture of these or not identify with any of them but still want to experience a male-to-female makeover. For example, a female impersonator, stage performer, or drag queen. Maybe you are gender fluid, non-binary, or have a bit of both and are looking for ways to combine masculine and feminine traits. Perhaps you are just beginning to realise that this is something you want to explore. Let's talk about that for a moment.

Why do I feel like this?

Women learn how to be feminine through socialization. Girls and women internalize these 'acceptable' feminine traits and social behaviours. The typical way this occurs is by being rewarded in some way for what might be called gender appropriate behaviour. The same applies to boys and men except that female traits are discouraged while masculine traits are reinforced.

This process of socialization leads to the extremes of the girly girl and the manly man. But, of course, there is a whole spectrum in between. In this book we want to help you find your own place on the scale and feel comfortable with yourself and how you express your own femininity.

Here is a list of five possible scenarios that may have contributed to your feelings and desires.

Female household: You were brought up in a dominantly female household. In this case the family structure might have been very matriarchal with wives, aunts, sisters and female life being the main focus with men in the minority or on the periphery. In this case you may have seen feminine behaviour has more 'normal' and were socialised more than the average male towards female behaviour and dress. That doesn't mean that you like to dress all the time or even at all but are more sensitive to the idea of feminine things and behaviours.

Male Household: in this case you lived in a patriarchal household where the dominant characters were male and you identify with female roles for several reasons. If you had sisters that were 'Daddies favourite' you may have felt left out and unconsciously been envious or jealous and formed a view that femininity was a way to get love and attention. Alternatively, your male role models may have been domineering and boorish especially when it came to women and you concluded that you didn't want to be like that.

Inner balance: Alternatively, your inner balance of female or male energy is simply such that you identify more with the feminine than the male. If this develops you may become unhappy or depressed that you are not who you want to be or that you cannot express yourself fully in public. The idea of being in the wrong body (or body dysmorphia) is very complex and not something we can deal with here. If this sounds like you then please look at the transgendered resources locally or on the internet. They will be able to support you in finding out who you really are. Then when you need help dressing and being feminine come back and look at the ideas in these pages.

The thrill: Another reason for dressing is that you find it all a little naughty and exciting. Usually this is because you have somehow developed a fetish for female things. There can be a whole bunch of triggers here. Maybe you liked the softness or silky feel of garments when you had a cuddle from a female carer or perhaps you had a comforter made of a satin or lacy slip when younger. Perhaps you envied little girls who could wear pretty party dresses. Maybe you played harmless dress up with sisters and other girls when you were very young. Perhaps your mom or auntie dressed you in girl clothes or pants when your clothes got messed up and they didn't have anything else at hand. Or perhaps you just got a thrill from trying on lingerie and underclothes when you were left alone in the house.

Abuse: And finally, we have to mention the fact that you may have been mistreated when you were growing up. No one likes a reminder of this but sometimes dressing in adult life can be a form of acting out. Dressing for erotic reasons is not considered a mental health condition if it does not cause distress. Technically though if a person indulges in crossdressing for purposes of sexual excitement for a period extending beyond six months and it causes distress or impairment to the individual it is classed as a mental disorder.

We don't condone any form of sexual abuse or non-consensual activities in this book. If this has happened to you please please arrange to see a counsellor and/or report people to the authorities. There are lots of helplines and other on-line resources that can start the process. Get all that sorted and then if you are still interested in dressing and being feminine read on.

So, there can be very complex reasons why people want to crossdress. Some people worry that wanting to dress is a latent desire to be gay. The vast majority of men that like to dress and enjoy girl time are heterosexual. And, if you are in transition or identify with a gender different from the one assigned at your birth then is it really crossdressing at all? Of course, it doesn't matter what your orientation is for you to enjoy feminization.

Do you have a look?

Now before we get too maudlin let's spend some time figuring out what you want. If you don't have a 'look' yet it is worth taking a few moments to think about what you find attractive about women in general. Who do you want to be like? Spend some time looking through women's magazines and the fashion pages. What do you like on TV or in movies? What is your favourite genre? How do the women dress? How do they do their makeup and hair? How do they act? Don't worry about whether it is realistic for you we will get to all that later.

If you find yourself admiring a woman in the street or in a restaurant what do you like about her? A good indicator that you are ready for your makeover is when you stop thinking whether you have a chance with her and start wondering where she got her clothes from, who her stylist is, and what it would be like to be her. You might admire the way she sits and holds herself. It can be little things like the way she dabs her lipstick after eating or drinking, plays with our touches her hair, or something more mundane like how she wears a t-shirt, jumper or a blouse. Maybe you like how she shows off her legs or the kind of stockings or shoes she wears. You'll feel something inside – that says, yes, I want to be like her.

For simplicity we can consider three basic looks that, as it turns out, align themselves with the three phases of feminism. The first wave occurred in the late 19th and early 20th century with an emphasis on legal issues and rights. This was the era of the suffragettes and ended roughly with women gaining the right to vote. Before that however women had few rights, could not own land or inherit wealth, and often were regarded as possessions. Think of Jane Austen novels where women were left penniless and homeless and without status when widowed or without a man or husband to support them.

If you enjoy a female led relationship or are being feminized by a partner, you might also subscribe to some of these values or roles. You might even like to indulge in period costume. For example, an empire style dress, southern belle or a restrictive Victorian garb. Let's be careful though we are not saying that you give up your rights to choose or to be free. Everything must remain consensual even if you want to be passive or submissive to your partner.

The second wave of feminism was not just about freedom and rights. Starting in the united states in the early 1960s it quickly spread across the western world. Second wavers asserted that girls were socialized with toys, games, television and school to adopt feminine behaviours. The cultural stereotype was that women were often childlike, dependent, and passive. The emphasis in the second wave was to undo this kind of Stepford wives programming to give women equality and to question the standards of female beauty at the time which objectified and subjugated women to assigned roles as wives, mothers, or sexual dolls.

To see how this depiction of women translates into expectation it is useful to watch films or look at advertising during the 1950s, 60s and 70s and notice how the clothing, style, and depiction of women changes. If you are attracted to any of these ideas then you might like a retro-style look and persona. For example, the smooth figure-hugging clothes in the TV series the Mad-Men or that Doris Day look with full skirts and petticoats typical of the 1950s and 60s. You might also like evening gowns or cocktail dresses.

The third wave of feminism takes a more balanced approach. With equality came the argument that traditional symbols of feminine culture should not be devalued. It recognises that while in the previous waves women often had no choice. In a modern setting feminine identity such as motherhood, stay at home wives, make-up, suggestive clothing, and sensuality can also be personal affirmations. As such a conscious decision to celebrate one's femininity can be a personal and empowering choice. So here we include the current trends for very short and revealing clothing, bodycon dresses, burlesque style, bimbos, and sluts. You might also think of yourself as a Barbie-girl.

Before you bridle at some of these labels a quick note on so-called 'lipstick' feminists. That was originally meant as a disparaging term but has actually turned out to be self-affirming. The thing that is affirmed is the right of a person to choose how they act and dress, not to be dictated to by some social convention. When we talk about bimbos and sluts we are using the words as a shorthand of accepted behaviour and societal expectations. Nice girls do not dress provocatively or act in sexually promiscuous ways. If your look leans towards the more salacious then be aware that this is the projection you will make to other people and they will treat you accordingly. Likewise, if you want to be a 'good' girl and dress conventionally, nerdy, preppy or like Sunday school that is okay too.

Petticoating and Sissy play

Petticoating is the practice of feminizing boys or men for disciplinary reasons. In the past boys could be petticoated (or pinafored) for unruly behaviour, being curious about female things, teasing girls or disrespecting women. Boys would be made to wear dresses and do girl chores or be taken into town by mother for shopping and so forth. Sometimes the boy would be dressed identically to the mother or his sisters. The idea was that the humiliation of the experience would provide a strong incentive for a boy not to act in inappropriate ways. Of course, it is not rocket science to figure out that this is a very dubious practice and open to abuse where minors are concerned.

Adult petticoating remains a legal activity in many places provided it does not cause a public disturbance or involve obscene behaviour. In female led relationships or in some mistress led role play games an adult male is subject to a feminization fantasy. The person is 'forced' to undergo feminization under the threat of corporal punishment, public or erotic humiliation (whether it is actual or implied.) Often this involves being made to wear female lingerie under ordinary male clothes, dressing as maids and doing chores, or being made into sissy girls that play with dollies or carry a purse. Of course, this mimics the idea of female socialisation. In these circumstances the male enjoys the feelings of submission, embarrassment and control. And, quite often develops more feminine attributes over time.

We mention petticoating here because it is a popular pastime for potential crossdressers and the genre itself has quite a significant following in fictional literature. Because of the requirements for humiliation the types of feminization are quite specific. The clothes worn also involve very elaborate frilly and short dresses that you wouldn't ordinarily see an adult female wearing. If you are attracted to this kind of thing then there are a number of genre specific web suppliers. We don't cover any of this in detail but the process we follow for feminization can be adapted to role play directed by a partner. We will also cover all the types of cuts and materials for clothes so you know what kind of pretty things you like.

What do you want to achieve?

After all that now is also a good time to think about your objectives. Usually dabbling with clothes and makeup and being girly for a while is done behind closed doors. It can be a solitary affair. You might also chat on-line with like-minded people and you might even enjoy skype or camming and want to perfect your look for that. If you are brave you may want to venture out to friendly clubs, go to the movies, or shopping at the mall. You might also want to prepare to come out to your close friends or develop sufficient confidence to dress for work as part of your transition. In this sense an objective is to be 'passable'.

That's a horrible phrase but what it means is that when you go out in public people don't give you a second glance. You pass as female. This doesn't necessarily mean that you are bombshell gorgeous. No, what we mean by passable is that your ensemble works. That things like hair and make-up don't give you away. That you know how to deport yourself – such as walking properly in heels or sitting properly. That other women don't look at you and see a fashion disaster. In short that you don't give yourself away by a 'tell'. Something that stops people and makes them ask – 'is she?'

Of course, when you bring all the factors together and create that mystique of the feminine, people may still look at you. They may secretly admire your elegance and grace. There are many cross-dressers, tgirls and trans-girls that put catwalk models to shame. If someone does share your secret then the person will do a double take and say 'no, I don't believe you – are you sure.' That's what passable means. If all that sounds too daunting right now, it is still worth putting time and effort into the detail so that your own private time can be just as rewarding. Even if you just want to take selfies or potter about in your own home. Remember it is not just about the look but also how you feel. How at ease you are with your inner self.

Makeover Experiences

If you are lucky then you might have some other girl friends that you can share experiences with. A surprising number of women, wives, and girlfriends find they have a curiosity or will help someone like you explore their other side. If nothing else girly girls like playing dress up, doing hair, and makeup. If you have someone sympathetic, great, they will help you with many of the topics in this book. It can be fun to explore together.

If you are a singleton then you can still have some interaction by booking a makeover appointment. Normally these services are run by sympathetic females, transgender women, or other crossdressers. You sign up for a day or afternoon and they will feminize you. This involves hair and makeup plus a number of outfits. Once dressed you can socialise en-femme or be a model in a photoshoot where a professional photographer will take pictures for you to keep as a memento or to use in your web pages or blogs.

By and large these services are very discreet. Often the organisers have been where you are and appreciate what it takes for you to take such a step. For extra safety, check if their services are listed or mentioned on crossdressing friendly forums and sites. What do the members have to say about them?

If the idea of a makeover appeals to you then here are a few things to think about. First check out the testimonials and galleries (some visitors will allow their pictures to be used) – this will let you know how friendly and competent the people offering the makeover are. Look at the style of the make up in the examples – is it every day or more drag queen. What kind of wardrobe do they have; extensive or small, in a variety of sizes and cuts, and do they carry a range of 'man' sized (bigger) women's shoes. Sometimes they will hold clothes that it would be uneconomic for you to buy yourself. For example, bridal outfits, prom dresses, sparkling cocktail or party dresses, as well as some period costumes like southern belle or even princess or quince dresses.

In booking an appointment the person will want to know your girl sizes and the kind of 'look' you want to experience. This helps them get a selection of outfits and hair pieces ready for you and allows them to plan the day. In some cases, they will let you bring your own things, but you need to ask. Also, they may do 'sissy' dressing but don't expect them to play the role of a mistress. There are other professional services for that. And you'll probably offend the person and they will not book your session or respond to further contact with you. They also expect that you will have made an effort to look femme. For example, they won't do shaving, hair removal or other hygiene on the day so you must have got yourself appropriately ready beforehand.

When the people get to know you (several visits) they may also be happy to accompany you on a shopping trip or afternoon out, and may even introduce you to other 'girls', or arrange a 'girls' night out at a crossdressing friendly venue. Sometimes they will do make-and-go where you can have your makeup done for a night out yourself (with your own clothes), offer bed and breakfast, or other forms of social event. The more established places will also offer feminizing products and makeup to purchase. And, if your femme side is a secret, they may offer locker facilities for you to store your stuff.

If you are intrigued by the above but struggling to answer any of the questions about what you want, then you are probably not ready for a makeover service just yet. Reading this book will help clarify the things that you do want and the things that you don't. The more honest you are the better your experience will be. Also, you'll appreciate the kind of things you might want to purchase – it's not just about wigs and makeup.

About the book

Whatever your reasons for reading, the real you, the girl inside, will have some ideas on the way she wants to be. She may surprise you. Go with her and realise her ambitions. Each chapter gives some insight and some things to develop and practice. Some of this is generic some is more specific and detailed. We also give you a shopping list for the things you need at each stage.

An assumption is that you were not socialised as a girl. As a result, we need to revisit and spend time on all the little things females seem to find so natural and take for granted. Getting in touch with your femininity is a mixture. An ensemble if you will of lots of things. When you see an ultra-feminine woman, the way she acts and dresses, the way she walks and talks, and oozes sensuality you know there is something more going on than just putting on a dress.

Part I considers what you want to achieve with your girl time. We look at what makes us physically one sex or another and how flexible and open this is to change. Then we move onto how to treat your body right and indulge in all those little things that make a woman feminine.

In Part 2 we go on to consider ways to sculpt or contour your body so that it remains in proportion but more idealistically female. We look at boobs, butts, and tucking.

In Part 3 we move onto dressing the body. We consider the wonderful world of sexy lingerie and underwear and how the right materials and textures can give you that lovely feminine feel. Then we look at clothes and how the right cut and hang of materials as well as patterning and combinations can flatter your figure. And, finally, we consider movement and deportment. In particular, how to walk in those ultimate expressions of female sexuality your heels.

The chapters are presented in a particular order so that each one builds a foundation for the next. Of course, that doesn't mean that you cannot dress fully from day one just that you will get more competent as you develop each of your female attributes. If you feel drawn more to one part than another or feel you don't need one section that is fine. You can always refer back. In each section there are also a number of options. You may find that one way of doing things works better for you or you find it easier to accomplish your look by cherry picking bits from each part. That is fine as well.

Having said all that – if you are ready let's enter the boudoir.

Chapter 2 What makes us Male or female

In this chapter we explore how we can influence the natural instincts of the body to express itself. There is a bit of science here as the objective is to show how much of your body can be made more feminine by changing its chemical balance or via cosmetic procedures. Skip on to the next chapter if you aren't interested in why females are softer and rounder, how breasts grow, or muscles and fat develop.

A simple way to put this into context is by three basic levels of sex characteristics: primary, secondary, and tertiary. Primary sex characteristics are the ones that make someone male or female including the internal/external genitalia and sex organs. If you have testicles and produce sperm, you are male. If you have uterus and produce eggs, you are female. The other physical aspects we associate with being male or female, like breasts, curviness, and muscles are all secondary and are caused by hormonal changes as we grow. With a little help these secondary things can be changed. And with gender reassignment you can address the primaries as well.

The third set of characteristics are what we might call electives. Left to themselves the primary and secondary characteristics are controlled by the body. The electives are how we choose to emphasise or de-emphasise our sexuality for example how we dress and do our makeup and grow or style our hair. In this chapter we are interested in the non-electives. It is surprising the degree to which even those can be influenced. As we move onto the later chapters, we will begin to make more elective choices and provide temporary work arounds for primary and secondary features.

The effects of Puberty

Ironically, it seems we all started off as girls. If you look at the middle of your scrotum and the part from there to your anus there is often a slightly different coloured seam of skin that looks like a join. That is exactly what it is. The future labia in a girl came together and joined up to make a boy. If you explore further, you'll also find a sensitive area about the size of your thumb nail called the lion spot. It is like a little dimple under the skin half between front and back and is pleasurably sensitive to massage – the remnant of the possible vagina. The future clitoris and urethra also come together to make a penis. All that happened while you were in the womb. Once born the way we turn out depends mostly on how hormones change our bodies.

As adults we can all remember the time when our body went through a lot of changes. Some of these changes aren't as fixed as we think. Before puberty, apart from the primary sex characteristics, male and females are pretty similar in skeletal, muscle, and fat distribution. During puberty we go through five stages (sometimes called Tanner stages, after a child development expert). Stage one occurs around 8 years old in girls and 9-10 years in boys. There are no outwards changes but the brain starts to increase the production of a range of hormones. Stage 2 occurs around 9-11 in girls and 11 in boys. Both sexes start to develop some pubic hair and the sex organs begin to mature. It is the testicles (boys) and ovaries (girls) that generate most of the testosterone and estrogen used to change our bodies. Both boys and girls have a mix of these powerful hormones.

Girls convert most of their testosterone to a form of estrogen called estradiol which among other things helps breasts develop. From Stage 3 (12 for girls and 14 boys) onwards the physical changes become more dramatic and noticeable. Pubic and under arm hair develops. The breasts develop in girls to reach a final size after 4-6 years. Girls reach full development at around 18 while boys continue for another two years developing greater height and muscle tone as well as hair on the back, chest, and face.

During puberty the skeleton, muscles, and fat distribution in our bodies change. The female pelvis widens and flattens. It is rounder and larger than the male so that a baby can pass through during childbirth. The sacrum (back of the pelvis or tailbone) tips more towards the rear which can result in hip sway or the characteristic way women walk. The ribcage is smaller in women and the ribs are shaped differently to allow for the growth of a baby. And, the bones in the upper arms are slightly more angulated outward so that the lower arms are free to swing without catching on the wider hip bones and help with carrying a baby on the hip. This freer wider hand movement is also typical of the female gait. When we learn to walk like a woman, we'll have to remember these points. And when we choose female clothes because the rib cage is shaped slightly differently even if you choose the right size dress the zip or buttons often won't fasten properly at the back when the bodice is close fitting. As a result, you may need to go to a size bigger.

Usually, a woman has a low waist to hip ratio with the hips close to or beyond the shoulders. This leads to traditional view of women as having a smaller hourglass form. In contrast men have a narrow pelvis, wider ribcage, and shoulders. This leads to the traditional view of men as having triangular shaped upper bodies. If you take the size of your head from top to chin, on average the male shoulders are 2.5 heads wide compared to a woman who is 2 heads wide from shoulder to shoulder. Likewise, the average body is eight heads high but because the woman has a smaller head she is usually shorter than the male.

According to fashion designers the idea female height is 5'8"so a shorter female will add height by wearing heels. But if you are a male, heels can sometimes make you look excessively tall. Women typically are between 5',4" and 5', 6". This is the range that clothing manufacturers cater for. If you are a short male with a slight frame, you'll find female clothes fit more easily. If you are bigger framed, you will need the plus sizes.

Diet and Exercise

Unlike bone structures which are permanent once they are formed the degree of muscle and distribution of fat can vary depending on our hormone levels, diet, and exercise.

Testosterone helps build muscles through exercise. Because men have about ten times more testosterone than women, they bulk up more. Men develop muscles in the upper arms, chest area, and on the back of the upper legs. Women on the other hand tend to develop leaner muscles all-over but particularly on the front of the upper legs. You can see these differences by looking at male and female gymnasts. Male gymnastics is mostly about upper body strength and power. Female gymnastics is mostly about lower body strength and balance.

A woman has to exercise significantly more than a male counterpart to get the same level of muscular development, but it can be done. If you look at female cross-fit competitors, you will see similar upper body and abdominal development to males. The reverse is also true. If you want leaner more feminine muscles switch your exercise from a focus on resistance work (like lifting weights) and do more softer stretching and strength activities like Yoga and Pilates.

In your socialisation into female behaviour it won't take long to realise that women talk about diet and exercise quite a lot and seem to always be on one regime or another. There is a good reason for this. Women tend to retain more fat than men. Men burn fat more efficiently. Estrogen influences how fat is made and stored in the body, as a result women tend to store more fat than men. This extra fat is distributed throughout the body under the skin. Hence women generally have rounder limbs and softer faces. If you try and target an area for fat reduction with diet and exercise, you'll find that fat reduces all over your body not just the area you want. You might find you reach the right weight but that areas you wanted to tone up still look fat.

Estrogen causes more fat to be stored on the hips, buttocks, and thighs. Hence women look wider on the hips and upper legs. Younger females tend to be lithe, so body contoured and tight-fitting clothes look fantastic on them. Men, with lower estrogen, tend to develop fat on the stomach. When a woman gets older and reaches menopause the estrogen levels drop and more fat is deposited on the stomach area just like a man. Thus, as women age, they tend to look more like men in shape. This is good news if you are a middle-aged or mature crossdresser. Assuming, of course, that you dress age appropriate.

Three Basic body types

Your bone density, fat, and muscle definition can be used to define three basic types of body. We'll look at more body types in chapter 4 where the emphasis will be on proportion. First though, are you an endomorph, mesomorph, or ectomorph?

Ectomorphs are long and lean looking. They have a delicate frame similar to marathon or long-distance runners. Typically, they have fast metabolism. They process food quickly and burn energy fast, so they are what are called hard gainers. That is, they find it difficult to put on weight or fat no matter how much they eat and can take a higher carb diet than the other two types. Typically, these females will look great in anything that outlines the figure or contour and shows off long legs. However, they can also come across real skinny so lingerie and slinky bedroom attire might not work for them. A male ecto will want to emulate how a female ecto dresses to get the best look.

Endomorphs are stocky in build and have wider bodies. They have more muscle than Ectos but the downside is they have more fat too. Excess food is stored as muscle and fat in the lower half of the body, so they tend to have big butts or thighs. Their metabolism is slow, so they find it difficult to stay lean or trim looking and benefit from high intensity workouts. In short, they are what we call hard losers because fat stays on the body. Diet wise they should reduce carbs and increase protein. They also tend to need their sleep and put weight on when they are stressed. Because of the heavier build, things like tight fitting bodices, frilly edges and puff sleeves, will make an endo look chunky. Looser clothing and things that make you look taller is the way to go. Stockings and heels will make you look chunky but lovely diaphanous babydolls and/or negligees will give a sensual edge. If the figure is on the curvier side, you'll look voluptuous.

Mesomorphs are the inbetweeners. They can be both lean and muscular at the same time. Often, they are natural athletes like gymnasts or multi-eventers. Mesos have that middle of the road body. They find it easier to lose weight than Endos and build muscle easier than an Ecto. As a Meso you can exercise moderately and still control your weight and fitness. A female meso might have that tomboy or the girl-next-door look and can look pretty in just about anything. The balance of fat to muscle means they look healthy but are also curvy as well. Because a Meso looks fit they can get away with just about anything in the lingerie department and can choose tight or flowing dresses.

A few takeaways from this section. If you are a woman and want to show more muscle development don't work as hard in the gym but do lose fat – that way your existing muscle will show up more. Likewise, if you are a man stop doing the heavy workouts and switch to gentler stretching exercises which build strong, flexible, but lean muscle. That way your musculature will be more feminine. Be careful though, you cannot target or spot-tone an area. Your body will lose or gain fat all over no matter what your focus is. People have certain areas that are prone to development or reduction. In men extra fat heads for the stomach in women it goes for the hips and buttocks. How much you get and where depends on your predisposition as an Ecto, Endo, or Meso. Later we'll show you how to overcome some of these leanings and dress right for your body type.

Breast development

Next a little word about breasts. We have a whole chapter on creating a realistic bust later on but estrogen levels also affect breast development.

Breasts start to develop in girls at stage 2 of puberty as a result of estradiol. They start with budding which makes the future nipple area sensitive and itchy. Then as more fat is deposited the ducting and mammary glands develop to bulk up the shape of the breast (see Figure 5 in Chapter 5.) Boys also have low levels of estrogen which they make by converting testosterone to estradiol. They also have the latent ducting and glands. Hence some boys will also develop breast tissue in puberty until the balance in testosterone evens out. As men age their testosterone levels drop and this can lead to fat deposits, hair loss and reduced muscle definition. The higher proportion of estrogen may also trigger breast development. If the hormones fail to balance sufficiently it can lead to a condition known as Gynecomastia (or man-boobs).

Breast tissue is not muscle. The breast sits on top of the pectoral muscles. Although there is some fat in their most of the bulk is the mammary glands designed to supply milk to the nipple. If you think you may have man-boobs a quick check is to gently press around the nipple area. Is there a small lumpy feel that shows duct and gland development? Also, you might see a darkening of skin around the nipple which are called areolae. The area might also be sensitive and itchy. If there is nothing under the nipple then it's just excess fat (sorry!) By the way if you do feel some lumps or you have discharge from the nipple or are itchy best to get a check-up with your doctor just to be on the safe side and rule out anything more sinister.

If you are a small breasted female (or trans-girl) you can increase your bust size a little by exercising your pectoral muscles to bulk them up. A good exercise for this is to hold your arms out in front of your chest, bend the elbows so you can touch your palms together, and then push them against one another. This will exercise the muscles and also give you an idea of how much fat is above. Another popular exercise is to do push ups or exercise with small dumb bells (one for each hand) and bring your arms together and then out to the sides. Do this exercise regularly (20-30 reps per day) and you'll firm up and add some bulk to your existing boobs.

Another thing to note is that depending on your basic body type you'll need to think about the size of your boobs. Ectomorphs are lean and tall, so their chests are smaller relative to height meaning they have proportionally smaller boobs. Endomorphs are chunkier and wider so the boobs tend to be more substantial. And, Mesomorphs, are like goldilocks, their boobs are neither two small nor too large. Of course, we are only talking averages, some people will be bigger chested than their type and this will make them more busty looking while others will be smaller chested for their type and look more boyish. If you are aware of these simple body types though you can see when a girl is oversize for her type or where the cosmetic surgery has been overdone.

The takeaway is to think carefully about your body type before you decide how big you want to be. If you choose a breast size relative to your body type you will be much more passable. More on this in later chapters.

A second Puberty

Although you cannot change your primary sex characteristics and the bone structure without some kind of surgery, we can alter the secondary characteristics by changing the balance of testosterone and estrogen in the body. This is why hormone treatment is effective for male to female transition.

Increased levels of estrogen in the body will change the way you store fat and that will make you look more female. A carefully supervised Hormone replacement strategy inhibits the production of testosterone and boosts estrogen. It doesn't happen overnight though. Just like your first puberty it can take the body a few years to get the levels right and make the changes.

You might think that upping your level of estrogen is therefore a good way to get proper boobs and a more femme look for free. There are all sorts of articles about how to increase your breast size by eating estrogen rich foods like lentils, yams, and soya. What we are talking about here are phytoestrogens which are plant versions of estrogen which the body recognises and will absorb. These are already in our diet so to make any difference you'd have to eat a lot of stuff- way above the daily dosage to have any effect. In one study women went on a yam rich diet for 30 days and did show improved estrogen levels.

You may also find a range of breast enhancement creams which again contain an array of firming agents and plant extracts. Natural oils such as Almond, Olive, Jojoba, Coconut, Lavender, Emu, Primrose, Flaxseed and so on contain fatty acids and vitamins that the body absorbs and can help bulk up your breast tissue. Rub them into the breast area everyday working out from the nipple area. The massaging improves circulation while the fatty acids and oils add volume to your breasts. Obviously, they work better if you have some material to work with and bulk up.

A note of caution though. It is not all about estrogen. Other hormones such as prolactin, and progesterone and growth hormones are also important. If your estrogen spikes or passes a threshold compared to other hormones you become what is called estrogen dominant. This is an indicator for all sorts of illnesses and complications including heart disease and cancer. If you have had any health conditions that are hormone related (like prostate problems) then you need to be careful. Higher estrogen may also affect your mood, lower your sex drive, shrink your male bits, and/or lead to erectile dysfunction. If any of these are important to you then don't mess with your estrogen levels.

If you do want to grow your breasts or look naturally more female it is worth seeing a hormone replacement specialist and talking to someone who knows how to handle the changing balances and what symptoms to look for. They can change your regime or indeed advise you of any contraindications in your medical history. Again, this all costs money and if you want any chance of doing it on medical insurance or as part of a free health programme you will have to consider some counselling and talk to people about gender transitioning before you will be seriously entertained. It is a complicated legal minefield and the procedures are often considered elective or cosmetic. The risks and possible side-effects make insurers extra cautious.

Informed Consent

Today there are many more possible cosmetic procedures from breast implants, fillers, liposuction, butt lifts, tummy tucks, and all kinds of techniques to alter your face. If you decide you like your look and want to permanently transition, then the above can change your shape permanently. Such a decision is indeed a serious step and not to be taken lightly.

Once you start on this journey it can be fulfilling and rewarding and may well complete you. But, it will alter your relationship with family, friends, and at work. In the following pages we will show you how to get the same effects without invasive cosmetic procedures.

Years ago, it was virtually impossible to embark on permanent feminization without having a referral to a psychologist. This is still true if you want to opt for the ultimate procedure to change your primary sex characteristics. You may need to spend a significant time living 24/7 and holding down a job as a female before you can be a candidate for surgery.

For secondary sex characteristics, in most countries where this is possible, the regulations have relaxed considerably. Often these things are considered a lifestyle choice and many cosmetic surgeons or doctors will act on the principle of informed consent. That means that as long as they are convinced that you are mentally stable, capable of understanding what you are doing, and the likely consequences then you are a candidate for a procedure.

Of course, none of this will be relevant to you if all you want is some girly playtime. But if you are beginning to spend more time in your female persona it is something to think about. Use the rest of this book to develop your look and find out what changes you want to make so that you are indeed informed when or if you want to take things further. And whatever your decision. Good luck.

Chapter 3 How to Pamper your body

This chapter has three main purposes. First is to give you all the information you need about looking after your skin. Second is to give you some practical advice on removing that unsightly male body hair and maintaining a more feminine look. And third is to give you some self-indulgent pampering so you can enjoy your body in a female way.

We will also throw in a few tips about things like pheromones and nails. Your body odour sends chemical signals that marks you as male. Likewise, poor nail care and style is one of the most obvious 'tells' that you are not female. We'll give you some solutions that work whether you are a permanent or occasional crossdresser.

Now, first off is skin. When we start to think about different dress styles it is obvious that we will expose different areas of the body. Females generally tend to show more of their body than males. We need to think about how we appear when we expose more of our skin. If we are taping or wearing foundation garments (see later) to create a feminine look we will also want to take care of our more sensitive areas properly. And, finally, but definitely not least, is that feminine feeling of being smooth and enjoying the brush of soft and silky fabrics. Each of these things is an important part of your socialisation as female.

Even if you don't dress frequently there is no reason why you cannot enjoy a feminine lifestyle. You can do these pampering routines right alongside your day-to-day existence. No one would ever suspect. And, it will make your dressing so much more enjoyable. It will also give you something to talk about with your other 'girl' friends. Go on, indulge your inner self. You're worth it!

Skincare

Soft skin is very feminine and when looked after properly takes on a nice healthy sheen and glow. The two key points here are cleanliness and moisturising. Both these things can be achieved by regular showering or bathing. Apart from the functional process of washing treat yourself to a couple of indulgent sessions a week. Pamper yourself by buying products that have a pleasant (feminine) smell and or the dual effect of relaxing your muscles and body. Regularly using an underarm deodorant with a neutral scent can also help to mask those busy male sweat glands.

Body odour occurs when bacteria on our skin break down sweat into acids. It can be an unpleasant smell if not attended to regularly and male and females smell different. Our sweat also contains pheromones which are chemical messengers that get emitted all over the body. Pheromones come in two types. One (the signaller) that acts as an attracter or repellent and is short acting. And, another (the primer), which produces changes in behaviour and increases hormone production in other people. Women are more sensitive than men when it comes to odour detection and can use it to get an unconscious feeling about sexual compatibility, health, or fitness, of a person and even menstrual cycles in other females. Females rely more heavily on these cues than men who depend to a greater degree on visual cues.

Perfumes and scented bodywashes can erase your natural scent and so remove your male cues. Most perfumes use musk compounds which are animal products with a similar chemical profile to our own body scents. Diet also affects how we smell. Women use both these methods to control body odour and so increase their sexual attractiveness. Jasmine is an aphrodisiac to both men and women. Lavender when combined with floral oils and cedar is attractive to men. Ylang ylang increases libido and Citrus increases energy. Vanilla, Orange, Pumpkin and Black Liquorice also attract males and females. In addition, women are attracted to smells such as lime, mint, ripe banana, chocolate, cucumber, and baby powder. Think about this when you are choosing your bubble bath, soak, or talc. Especially if it is just before you dress and/or go out.

Talcum powder can be used to alleviate any chafing from your foundation wear but also-absorbs excessive skin oils and picks up flakes of skin or other materials. A liberal dusting will also make your skin very smooth and smell attractive. Talc has had a bit of a bad press recently with women due to the assertion that dusting down below can lead to ovarian cancer. The reason for this is that some talcs contain traces of asbestos. Men are also inclined to lightly dust their bits. At the time of writing there have been no reported male cancers linked to talc. The sensible thing is to not use it excessively on your genitals or find more natural products instead.

Hydration and Moisturising

The second reason we want to pay attention to our skin is hydration and moisturising. The skin contains both water and oils (sebum) to maintain good health. When skin becomes dehydrated it can get dry and flaky, so we use hydration to improve the water levels. In moisturizing we attempt to improve the skins ability to retain water by maintaining the right level of oil. For a soft and smooth skin we need to both moisturise and hydrate. We can do this when showering or bathing by adding moisturiser to our shower or bath products. We don't want to overdo it though because then we get too much oil this can block pores in the skin causing spots and other irritations. Too much hydration can make you look fatter and your skin will get lazy and not produce enough hydrating material.

Men and women also differ in the amount of water they retain and the oil they produce. Men produce more of each so tend to have more oily skin. Women tend to lose oils and water especially as they age so they need more products in these areas. You might find that you don't have to do as much as your female friends to maintain healthy skin. Moisturizers come with different skin types because we all have different balances of oil and Ph (or acid levels) in our skin. Find out which one is right for you.

Male and female also differ in their approach to skincare. Women are happier to apply multiple layers of products to get that end result. Men though tend not to want to do this and will use multi-function products and things that are less oily. Hence our use of the term pamper yourself. Put aside some time and enjoy your pamper routine. Use aromatic oils or candles to set a nice feminine atmosphere and relax mentally as well as physically.

Exfoliation

The third skincare tool is exfoliation. Your skin naturally sheds dead skin cells to make room for new ones. For a typical cell this happens about every 30 days or so. These dead cells drop off and end up as household dust. However, the body is not perfect at shedding and our clothes compress areas so some cells can get stuck to the body. Excess cells are the cause of rough and uneven skin, can trap impurities and block pores to cause spots and other problems such as ingrown hairs.

Exfoliation is the process of removing these hangers-on by using granules, chemicals, or a tool. This allows moisturisers to penetrate the skin more deeply and make them more effective. It will also make your skin look fresher and healthier by improving skin circulation. It is a good idea to add exfoliation to your pamper routine. Whereas you can moisturise daily it is better to exfoliate only one or twice a week unless you have very oily skin in which case you need to do more.

Depilation

Armed with our skincare tools it is now time to turn to the important topic of hair removal (or to give its proper name – depilation.) Depilation is seen as a very feminine thing. Virtually all women engage in hair removal to some degree or another. Men are also becoming more interested in man-scaping which involves removal or trimming of body hair for cosmetic reasons. Men also shave their faces but we are assuming that as someone exploring feminization you are clean shaven and know what to do in that regard.

There are some basic differences between male and female hairiness that we picked up on in the previous chapter. In addition to the underarms and pubic areas, men have additional growth on the chest, shoulders, back, feet and hands. As a first step you might want to permanently remove these sections of hair. They are big areas, so your time on depilation is going to go up an order of magnitude compared to the average female if you keep them. Hair on your hands and feet are a giveaway because they are difficult to hide especially when you draw attention to them with nail polish and stockings. Women have arm and leg hair like men, but it is usually lighter and softer, so full arm hair removal is also a good idea. This will allow you to wear shorter sleeved outfits without any concerns.

This first step feminizes you back to the same degree of hair carried by the average woman and addresses difficult to reach areas and places that are going to show up when you wear female attire. With these areas gone you'll be free to dress whenever you want. Ideally, keep the under-arm, pubic, and leg hair. This makes your regime more traditionally feminine. Note though that many women regard hair removal as so onerous that they have these areas permanently removed as well. That would look odd for a man. If you ditch the obvious male areas and keep the rest that gives you something if you want to mix a feminine and male lifestyle.

With the above sorted you'll need a regular time to attend to your remaining needs. This involves depilating the legs, under-arms, and pubic areas. Men also tend to have more hair between the genitals and the anus (the peri-anal) region. The bottom cheek area may also need treatment as well. Because it is hard to reach this might be another area to consider for permanent removal especially if you are not very flexible. Also, as you get older it gets more difficult reach and to treat. Permanent hair removal methods often don't work on grey or white hairs so the sooner the better, darling.

Trimming down under

There are many pubic hair styles and you might want to think about feminizing yourself in this way. Note, though, that these styles are a little more difficult for the male to carry off because the pubic area doesn't end in a graceful Y shape. Here are the main female styles:

Bikini: a side trim of the pubes so you can wear smaller panties or indeed bikini bottoms. The hair at the sides and tops of your inner thigh are also removed.

French: Otherwise known as the landing strip. All hair is removed except for a small rectangle strip above the pubes. This makes it ideal for very skimpy panties like G-strings.

Brazilian: this is like the French style except that the shape is different. A Bermuda triangle points down towards the top of genital area. In the desert island the shape 'floats' on the pubic bone and leaves a gap to the pubic area.

Heart: is a variation on the Brazilian island style except the bit of fuzz left is shaped into a little heart (aw, so girly). Some people colour the hair and others have it shaped into other styles.

Hollywood: is so called because it is inspired by the porn industry in California. Basically, all the hair is removed from the pubic area. Currently this style is very popular among younger women.

Hollywood is a good choice for feminization because it clears the area for taping or tucking (see later). The heart or Brazilian is nicely effeminate if you are in a female led relationship or have a mistress that likes chastity and you don't want the device catching or snagging hair.

An alternative is to pretty up the male parts with a sissy pouch or sheath. This allows a more feminine shave as the male bits are hidden. Some people also tattoo the pubic zone with a motto, or a girly motif like flowers or butterflies. This can be hidden when the hair grows back. Not for everyone but plenty of choice.

Options for hair removal

There are many options for hair removal. Basically, though, it comes down to whether you want to shave them close, pull them out at the root, or destroy the hair follicle completely. The lighter options mean return hair growth and regular attendance. The heavier ones will stop hair growth or thin it out considerably. Here are your choices:

Shaving: exactly as it says. Cover the area with shaving foam or gel and apply the razor. Gives a close shave taking the hair close to the skin. Can lead to ingrowing hairs if not careful or you use a dull razor that pulls or drags the hair. Always use a disposal pack (buy the pink girly ones – they have a soothing strip). Relatively low pain but can be hard to reach some areas. A major advantage is that it can be applied to the genital areas so you might want to use other methods for larger areas and shaving for intimate bits. If you do shave the intimate parts use a gentle astringent like witch hazel to close up the pores afterwards. It stings like crazy for a moment, but you'll get less problems with itching, skin infection, spots and a smoother finish.

Waxing: here warm wax is painted over the area and covered with strips of paper. Once dried the paper is used to remove the wax which rips the hair out of the follicle. Very smooth finish and will last longer than shaving. It is more painful though. No gain without pain. Exfoliating and using talc beforehand can reduce this. Waxing can be done at home for small areas (like legs) but better to go to a salon for larger and difficult to reach areas. There are plenty of male salons if you are too embarrassed to go to a beauty parlour. Waxing cannot be applied direct to genitals, areas with large moles, or varicose veins but can be used to trim pubic hair.

Creams: a cream is rubbed over the area which reacts with keratin in the hair weakening it, so the hair falls out. After 5-10mins the cream can be washed (or scraped) off to leave a very smooth finish. Less painful than waxing and closer than shaving but have to get the coverage right. Cream cannot be applied to genital areas. It contains an ingredient that will be absorbed by the skin and can cause chemical castration amongst other complications. Likewise, will sting very badly and burn sensitive areas like the anus. Do a patch test to make sure you will not react to the chemicals in other places. Side-effects can include burns, rashes, and blisters. Since male hairs are generally thicker than female ones buy the male hair removal products to get going. Use the femme ones later, when things are more manageable and the hair is weaker.

Epilation: uses an electrical device called an epilator. The Epilator grabs the hairs and pulls them out in a similar way to waxing. Unlike waxing this does not pull skin cells off at the same time so theoretically less irritation. But again, not easy to use with difficult to reach areas and genital areas are out of bounds. Can also cause in-grown hairs. For the best results only use an epilator when the hair is short otherwise it can hurt like crazy. The hair may also get stuck in the mechanism if they are too long. Ow!

Permanent hair removal

For a more permanent solution the hair follicle from which the hair grows needs to be destroyed. Each hair grows in a cycle. A hair can be in one of three stages, growing, intermediate, or resting (or shedding). The first stage can last 3-5 years, the intermediate 1-2 weeks, and resting 3-4 months. Any treatment for permanent removal is going to have multiple visits (6-8) and take about 6 months to catch and kill all the resting hairs which could begin to grow again. Your three main options here are:

Electrolysis: a needle is placed into the hair follicle and short radio frequencies are used to kill it. Very effective and most often used for facial hair. This has to be done by a professional and can be costly with multiple visits so usually it is good only for small areas.

Laser: a laser delivers high heat down the hair to destroy the follicle. Tends to work best on people with lighter skin tone and darker hair. There are some medications which are contraindications and best not to tan or go out in the sun before treatments as this reduces effectiveness of the laser. Can be done as a beauty treatment with multiple visits but there are now some home applicators. The quality of the laser is important to the outcome. You get what you pay for.

Thermoelectric: Another popular home solution that claims to give spa-like results is the No-No device. Again, this works by delivering heat (via an electrical current) to remove the hair but also channels heat down the hair to inhibit growth in the follicle. Over time the follicle weakens. It gives a better result than an epilator because it is gentler and there is reduced possibility of an ingrown hair but it takes more time to get the same result as other methods. Patience is a female virtue.

Pre and post care

Whatever technique you choose there is some preparation and aftercare that is always worthwhile. Let's think about the process. To remove the hair causes disruption around the site of the hair follicle. Your skin can react to this and become sore. With the hair gone skin oils and dirt can get into the hole, blocking it up. And, depending on how the hair breaks off, when it starts to grow again it might grow flat and get stuck in the skin (an in-growing hair).

The best preparation for hair removal is to bathe in warm water to open the pores and to excise excess skin oils and dirt. Gently exfoliate the areas to remove any dead skin cells that might get pulled off in waxing or contribute to breaking hairs off in a way that will make them in-grow. If you are waxing later add some talc to soak up excess moisture so the wax strip sticks better to the hairs and the pull off won't hurt so much. If you are doing laser don't moisturise or use creams a day or so before your appointment. They will coat the hairs and make it more difficult for the laser to work.

For all the techniques make sure that the hairs aren't too long or short. Long enough to get a purchase on the hair is all that is needed. The best length is about 3-5mm (or 1/8 in). Whatever your preferred treatment method is going to be shave down for the first time and let the hair regrow to the right length for removal. Thereafter you should go through your routine once every two weeks for non-permanent removal and four to six weeks for salon or permanent techniques (until all the hair has gone). This makes it much less painful and onerous. If your hair is darker you might need to do this more often and if it is lighter less often. For example, if you get darker (grey) patches under your skin as the hair re-grows. Your skin will react most for the first time but not be as sensitive once you get going. Little but often. For this reason, it is sensible to maintain your routine even if you are an occasional dresser. Otherwise it will be like the first time every time.

Post hair removal it is essential to soothe the areas with a hydrating moisturiser. This will address any scrapes, burns, or other reactions till they clear up. Something like Aloe Vera is very effective at taking away heat and irritation. Apply liberally straight after and then as necessary. Avoid any hot showers or heavy physical activity that will cause sweating for a day or two as this will open up pores and increase the probability of clogging. For a couple of days after your session wear loose fitting clothing so that you don't irritate, chafe, or block the skin. If you can, wear softer looser female clothing. Ideally do your regime at the start of a weekend so you can float around your home with loose girly clothes and wear a nightdress to bed. For the pubic and associated areas, a loose pair of boxers or a silky pair of cami-knickers are ideal. The cool fabric will help take any heat out of the area.

If later, you suspect an in-grown (hard red bump) then exfoliate and loosen the skin with a moisturiser to soften and allow the hair to pop out. If that fails, then use a pair of tweezers to pull it out. Don't just hope it will go away – it won't. And once you have got one established it is likely to come back and be more difficult to deal with. If the hair gets really embedded a trip to a beauty therapist might be necessary or to the doctor if it gets infected.

By the way, if you are doing hair removal for a make-over appointment, a photo-shoot, or some other outing do it a few days before so that you have time for any reaction to die down. Red blotchy or bumpy skin is not a good look. If your skin is very sensitive to one technique try another till you find the right process for you. The first time is usually the worse. If you establish a pamper routine and soften your skin regularly things will get easier as it gets used to treatment.

Tanning

The purpose of this section is to alert you to the fact that your sun exposure may give your secret life away. If you live in a climate that has a reasonable amount of sunshine you'll have to think about tan lines. Also, if you are having your hair permanently removed using lasers it is best not to go out in the sun or use tanning products until the treatments are completed. The extra melanin (the stuff that gives skin its colour) reduces the targeting and effectiveness of the laser.

Some people think tan lines can be super sexy. Others hate them. Back in the 1970s girlie magazines were fond of shooting nudes with tan lines. Showing which bits get exposed to the sun and which stay under wraps is naughty and intimate. Seeing a model with the outline of her swimsuit or bra and panties etched on flesh remains a turn on for many men. On the other hand, if you like wearing different swimwear or tops then you'll end up with a patchwork of unsightly lines.

If you only dress occasionally, you'll find that your boy clothes leave tan lines too and that can spoil the effect. A T-shirt outline when you're wearing a sleeveless or sweetheart dress is not a good look. A boy-shorts outline when you want to wear skimpy panties or swimwear bursts the bubble. Likewise, if you dress and go out for an afternoon you might forget that you'll get girl tan lines. Nothing more embarrassing than your locker room friends or an unsuspecting partner seeing the outline of your girlie swimsuit or your low-cut top.

The solution to all this is simple – get an all-over tan! Whether it is out of the bottle or from a tanning studio. That way you will never face embarrassment or get caught out. Of course, if you are being feminized your partner might decide that girl tan lines are just what you need. You might even like the idea as a reminder just like wearing panties under your normal clothes. C'est la vie. Just remember to wear things that cover-up if your dressing is a secret.

Nails and Hands

One thing that we can all agree on is that manicured and painted nails are quintessentially feminine. Male and female hands differ in that women's hands are less stocky and the fingers are proportionally longer and more slender. The shape of the nails are also different. Male nails being wider and square whereas in a feminine hand the nail is narrow and tapered. This is something to emulate in your dressing because coarse rough hands are an easy giveaway.

If you do any kind of manual work then you are likely to have calloused, broken, or rough skin. If you do a lot of housework your hands might also be rough and the nails brittle from constantly wetting and drying or the effect of cleaners like bleaches and washing up liquid. If you have work hands, don't despair. Use a working hand cream to close cuts and use moisturiser every time you wash your hands till the softness improves.

As an off and on dresser you may think that hand care isn't important but if you have rough hands or jagged nails, you'll end up putting snags in your lovely delicate and silky outfits or laddering stockings. The same goes for toenails. If they are too long or rough, they will put holes in your stockings when you wear heels and all the pressure is downwards into the point of your toe. Likewise, if your heels have hard skin. A regular soak in the bath and use of a pumice stone to exfoliate the region can mitigate some of these effects.

Longer nails also require a different approach to handling things, opening, fastening and tying, and even using your mobile phone or typing on your laptop. If you are new to dressing and/or nails you might find it easier to put on your lingerie and stockings before you do your nails. These intimate garments have lots of fiddly catches and if you are not used to longer nails just getting dressed can be frustrating. Afterall, you don't want to break, pull off, or chip a nail!

All these things can serve as constant reminders of your femininity and so it is worth putting in some time and effort to have nice hands and nails. If you are being feminized or like sissy play a trip to the nail bar or salon can be expected. Also checking that your hands are neatly manicured and clean is a great source of disciplinary fun.

Figure 1 shows the most common female nail shapes. Notice that the ones at the left are passable male nails provided they are kept short. The ones to the right are more female with the pointed style extending to several kinds such a ballerina or coffin (tip of nail cut off) or stiletto (very pointed). The longer square nail with shiny shellac and a white tip is called a French nail and is very popular.

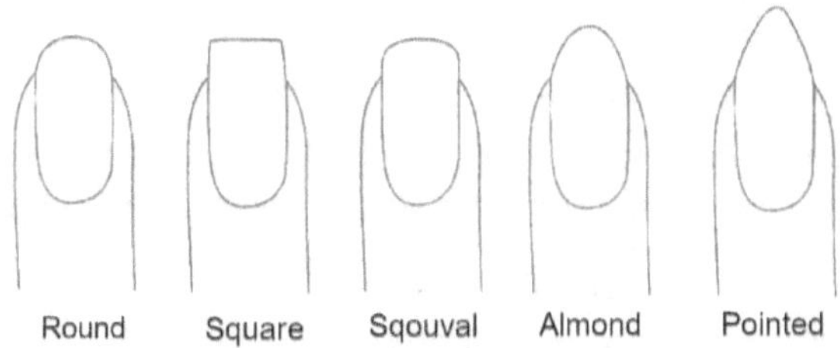

Figure 1 Common nail shapes

The good news is that you can have nice passable feminine hands that are also unobtrusive when you aren't dressed by following a simple regime. You don't need to go for cat-like talons or garish colours. Longer nails, nude and clear polish will make your fingers look thinner and hide the nail bed. Apparently amongst the British royal family women can only wear clear or nude coloured polish. So even with this simple approach you can still feel like a princess! If you want colour go for softer pinks, beiges, or olives that look more like natural nails.

If you do want brighter colours or longer nails for occasional use apply stick-ons. These are plastic nails that can be shaped and painted. All you need is to apply the sticky tabs provided or nail glue to your own nail and stick the pre-shaped nail onto it. The problem with these is that they tend to peel off and you don't want to be playing hunt-the-nail if your dressing is a secret. Glue ons are better but can be a devil to get off so the prep and removal time can impact on your girl time. This is especially important if you are time limited or dress while your partner is out.

A fashion trend at the moment is matte nail polish which is created by painting over the polish with a matte top-coat or by using baking soda or baby powder. The trick is to pour a little nail polish on a clean surface and then mix in small amounts of the powder. Make sure the polish is still spreadable even though it is thicker than usual.

You can also steam them. Heat a pan of water. Paint your nails as normal then hold your hands in the steam coming off the pan for 3-5 seconds, wiggling your fingers to get good coverage. It shouldn't affect the colour or the coverage of the polish but will dull the shine. A matte finish on clear or nude colours can be passable even when you are not dressed. Professional women that want neat but not obviously long nails will follow this routine and it won't draw attention in your workplace.

Creating soft feminine hands

Here is a six-step plan to keep your hands in lovely femme condition. If you follow the steps below you will grow better nails with more surface area to stick or glue onto or that you can paint quickly with coloured polish when you want to feel extra femme.

Step 1: *moisturise and exfoliate your hands regularly.* As we saw above the way to treat rough skin is to allow dead skin cells to come off the body. This also applies to the hands. We come into contact with lots of rough things. We also wash our hands regularly for hygiene purposes and also get them wet when we do household or other jobs. All this activity takes its toll washing out the oils so that the skin gets rough and breaks. Make sure you have some nice moisturizing hand lotion by the sink or in your bag. When you wash your hands and dry them add some lotion making sure you work it into the web of your fingers and also where the edges of the nail go into the skin.

Step 2: *keep your nails trimmed.* Nails grow at different rates and some get broken. When you see that they are uneven trim them back with nail scissors or a clipper. Make sure you are gently rounding the nail so that it takes on a more oval shape. How long you let them get is up to you. But longer ones will be more obvious and break more easily. Use a nail file to trim off any rough edges so that they are always smooth. This will avoid snagging your femme clothes.

Step 3: *strengthen the new growth.* A simple way to do this is to tap your fingers gently on a hard surface like a table (drumming your fingers). Foods that can improve your nails are fruits, lean meats, salmon, leafy green vegetables, beans and eggs, or nuts and whole grains. Alternatively use a hand cream that contains Royal Jelly.

Step 4: *give yourself a pedicure.* Trim your nails back every month or so (depending on how fast they grow) and shape them. In addition, soak your hands in warm water and moisturising soap. Then clean them removing any dirt under the nails that might attract fungus or infection. Use a soft brush to clean them up and then buff the nails. Next soak your hands in baby oil (or some other lotion with vitamin E) to keep them soft.

Step 5: *take care of your cuticles.* The cuticle is a sliver of soft skin at the bottom of your nail (or nail bed). The job of the cuticle is to stop bacteria sneaking into you via the join between the skin and nail. When this area gets dry or cracked you can catch and pull skin at the base of the finger plate which then becomes sore and causes the cuticle to grow back thicker. Soaking as in step 4 will help prevent this but you should also push the cuticle skin back regularly (weekly) using a cuticle pusher. This will make the nail plate look longer and neaten up the nail bed. Never cut the cuticle this will lead to infections. If you get any hanging dead skin snip the protruding edge with nail clippers so it doesn't catch on anything. Try and moisturise your cuticles everyday with a cuticle oil or petroleum jelly.

Step 6 *limit your use of nail acetone polish remover:* although nails look lovely when painted the removers contain some harsh chemicals that can irritate the skin and make your nails brittle and dry. Acetone is one of the worst so avoid using it if you can. Most stores will carry both acetone and non-acetone removers just read the label. Nail polish is a lacquer and sticks to the nail. So it is advisable to apply a base coat before the polish to make removal easier. Alternative removers are toothpaste which contain ethyl acetate also found in polish remover. Perfume will also work. Spray a little on a tissue and rub it into the nail.

Now you have beautiful hands and nails. What else can you do to make your hands look slimmer. Well, just like showing a bit of leg to make your ankles look more slender wear clothes that don't cover your wrists. Add some pretty bangles or a loose bracelet to give the impression that this area is more delicate. And, avoid jewellery that pinches or is tight on the fingers which will make them look fat. Unfortunately, pretty dainty jewellery with thin ring bands will just emphasize that you have male hands so use chunky stones to do the opposite.

High maintenance

As you can see, being feminine is a high maintenance activity. Once you start indulging your feminine side it does tend to take over. You will also need to be committed to looking after your body, what you eat, and how you exercise if you want to get the best look you can. Your femme figure will become important and you'll need to put time aside to look after it even if you don't dress all the time.

Here is our first little shopping list of things mentioned above:

Scent and essential oils (or candles)
Suitable feminine perfume (to disguise your male body odour)
Skin Moisturizers (body and shower wash)
Deodorant and/or body spray (for that neutral clean smell)
Bubble bath or equivalent (for pamper and softer skin)
Exfoliating granules (and or pumice stone for hard skin)
Wax strips, hair removal creams, or Lady shave (for legs and small areas)
Home Laser/ No-No or salon sessions for permanent hair removal and top-up (for big areas)
Shaving gel and disposable razors (for under arm, genital, peri-anal, and bottom)
Talcum (or baby) powder (for silky skin and pre-depilation)
Skin soother (aloe vera/witchhazel for post shave recovery)
Tweezers (for managing in-grown hairs)
Hand creams
Nail scissors and clippers
Nail polish (nude or clear)
Nail matte top coat (baking soda or baby powder)
Nail file or board (for shaping and smoothing rough nails)
Nail Buffer
Cuticle pusher

Cuticle oil and or baby oil (for softer hands)
Cotton wool/buds to help apply the above

Now you can appreciate why the gift of a little hamper of goodies is such a good present for the girly girl. And we haven't even got to hair and make-up or even basic clothes yet!

And finally ...

Just so you know. Beauty products often contain female hormones such as estrogen and progesterone. The body has receptors for these all over the body so a cream rubbed into the skin can absorb the material. The way this works is like patches used for some vitamins or nicotine. Rub them on your skin and they will get absorbed. In the previous chapter we talked briefly about the role of these hormones in breast development and other things. With all those extra girl products you will be increasing your exposure. Choose products carefully if this is not what you want. And, always read the label.

There are three main things to watch out for: parabens, placental extracts, and UV screens. These contain what are referred to as environmental estrogen. Parabens are basically used as preservatives in low amounts in lots of products. Placental extracts include estrogen, estrone, and progesterone as contaminants and are found in shampoos, conditioners, moisturisers, astringents and body creams. UV screens are photo-stabilizers that are easily absorbed by the skin and are found in high quantities in many products not just sunscreen. They are in perfumes, hairsprays, shampoos, conditioners, styling gels, facial creams, foundation, moisturisers, lipstick, hand soaps, body wash, insect repellent, nail polish, nail polish remover, and shaving creams.

Women are also more prone to skin discolouration (Melasma) due to hormonal balances. Men can get it too but women account for 90% of cases. Mostly it affects the face and forearms and other areas exposed to the sun. The skin develops blotches that are darker than your normal skin tone. They can go away by themselves or might need treatment. Because this condition is so common in women some beauty products contain an ingredient to bleach the skin. If a product says to lighten or brighten the skin it probably means that it has a skin bleaching agent.

Part 2
The Body Beautiful

I'm in a body that disagrees with me
There are straight lines were curves should be
I look in a mirror and what do I see
There is a girl inside that wants to be me.

Chapter 4 Body Shapes and Sizes

In the next three chapters we are going to start work getting the right body shape. First, we will look at some more body types that are all about proportions and make suggestions on how you can get an ideal female look. Then we will consider your vital statistics and the role they play in the fashion industry. This will allow you to order the right clothes for your size so that they fit properly in all the right places.

Another contribution of this chapter is to introduce the idea of foundation wear and padding. Women have used these techniques for years to give themselves more curvy figures, so it makes sense to learn from the pros. We'll look at each type of shapewear and their uses so you can decide exactly what you need to get the shape you want. After that we will move onto boobs, butts, and other bits to complete your female profile.

Body Shape

Our little biology lesson in chapter 2 provides some useful information about body shape. If you look at how people develop, they fall into a small number of types depending on bone structure, fat distribution, and muscle tone. Given your type you will be chunky, lean, or athletic. But just because you might be big boned, skinny, or prone to carrying additional weight that doesn't mean that you cannot look feminine. What is important is that you maintain certain proportions.

For simplicity we can reduce that down to five basic body types covering both men and women. The literature has more, especially for women, but these extras are all finer distinctions on the categories below. For example, spoon is variant on pear, diamond a variant on apple, cello a variant on hourglass, strawberry a version of the inverted triangle. We also give you some percentages of the various body types in the general population. The numbers for women are taken from a 2005 study of 6000 women by Carolina State University.

Type 1: Inverted Triangle or Tarzan

(5% of males have this shape, virtually no women)

Examples: Angelina Jolie, Cindy Crawford, Charlize Theron, Fedricia Pellegrini, Giselle Bundchen

This is the most obviously recognizable male type but is also one of the rarest. Only 1 in 20 men have this athletic look. A more common variation is the rhomboid (male) or strawberry (female) where the triangular shape is cut off and you look more rectangular. Women with a strawberry shape have shoulders that are wider than their hips, see examples above. You will also see it if a woman is a fitness fanatic and has a lot of upper body development that creates a triangle towards the waist. It isn't as obvious as the male because a woman usually has smaller shoulder width and they hide it with appropriate cuts of clothing. That is a clue as to how to deal with this type but we can also use foundation wear and padding to reduce the triangular effect by widening the bottom half of our body.

Type 2: The Oval or Apple

(25% of males, 14% female)

Examples: Rebel Wilson, Jennifer Hudson, Elizabeth Hurley, Rosie O'Donnell

The apple is more rounded in the waist area. The waist is often larger than the hips or bust area. Men develop this when they have too much fat deposited in the stomach area. Women also develop it as they get older and fat moves from the hips and thighs. But females might also have this as a natural type where the waist is not that defined. This is also the most common shape for mature men. One in four males have this body type and it is relatively easy to give you a more feminine rectangular, strawberry or hourglass look with a corset of cincher.

Type 3: The Rectangle or Banana

(40% of males, 46% of females)

Examples: Nicole Kidman, Kate Hudson, Gwyneth Paltrow, Sienna Miller, Gwen Stefani

The rectangle is what it describes which is straight up and down like a banana or ruler. In female circles it is often called the boyish look. The shoulders, waist, and hips are roughly on the same vertical line. Before puberty kicks in we are all rectangles. That is why if you played dress-up when you were small you probably found it easy to wear your sister's dress and it seemed to fit in all the right places. You can see from the numbers that this still covers quite a lot of the population. And, that is good news for crossdressing because it is one of the easier shapes to feminize. If you are this type, you may also be a shorter male and have more delicate bone structure. It will be easier to get an elvish or petite pixie look.

Type 4: The Triangle or Pear

(14% of males, 20% female)

Examples: Kristin Davis, Kim Kardashian, Rihanna, Mischa Barton, Eva Longoria

In this body the hips are wider than both the waist and the shoulders or bust. It is a very common female pattern (1 in 5 women have it). A lot of weight is carried around the hips, butt, and upper legs. This is one of the reasons women want to shed weight off their hips so that they look more in proportion. Hence the popularity of liposuction to literally suck out the fat and sculpt the body. Men can also have a pear shape but it is not very common (just over 1 in 10). That is also good news because it one of the more difficult shapes to feminize effectively. Though good child-bearing hips is often seen as womanly. And, females of this type use fashion and clothing cuts to help hide the hips.

Type 5: The hourglass or Barbie

(virtually no males, 8% female)

Examples: Beyonce, Scarlett Johanssen, Kelly brook, Katherine Heigl, Dita Von Teese

This is the typical sensuous shape we associate with sexy women everywhere. The main characteristics are for your bust and hips to be more or less the same width but with the waist narrower than the hips. Ideally the ribcage just under the bust also tapers in towards the waist as do the hips. When the shape is more rounded on the bust and hips it is referred to as voluptuous. A cello shape has slightly smaller bust than hips but not enough to be a pear shape. A spoon shape is even more exaggerated. If the bust is substantial it can look out of proportion or barbie like.

How does this help us with feminization? One way to interpret these body types is that before puberty we are all type 3 and when the hormones take over men tend to be pushed towards type 1 and type 2 while women are pushed towards type 4 and type 5. Of course, diet, exercise, and metabolism might resist this movement so that we end up with an intermediate type. If you are a small-framed man you might find yourself naturally placed towards the rectangle and hour-glass end of the spectrum. If you are also in the 5'4"- 5'-6" range height wise, that is going to make your makeover much easier and more convincing because you'll fit into the range used by manufacturers of female clothing. Figure 2 summaries all the information above.

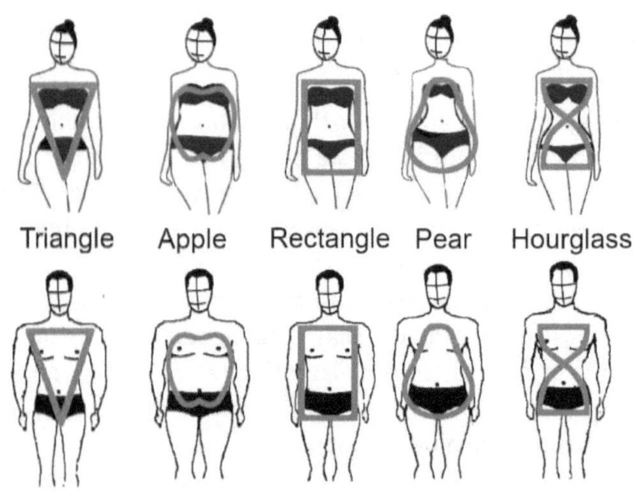

Figure 2 Different Body types

Your vital Statistics

So what type are you? Time to get the measuring tape out. Don't rely on your judgement or looking only in the mirror. That is often wrong because people see what they want to see. We need three measurements: bust, waist, and hips. As you measure pull the tape into an easy tension. The hips are the widest part just about level with but slightly above your crotch area. The waist is the narrowest part between the top of your hip bone and the bottom of the rib cage roughly in line with your tummy button. The bust line is around the curve of your chest muscles (or pecs).

A fourth measurement is the band. A line around your chest but under the bottom of where your breasts would be. The difference between the bust and the band give an idea of the breast size (or projection and fullness). There is also a letter associated with the bust size but more on that later. Right now, unless you are super flat-chested you'll have a little difference between bust and band because of any fat you are carrying on your chest or how developed the pecs are. So hey, we all have a breast size measurement.

These three measurements are what women refer to as their vital statistics. Usually it is vitally important that the middle number is smaller than the other two. If that is the case, then guess what. You are close to the ideal hourglass shape already and with a little help you can get a classy feminine look. The fashion industry and the expectations of society see the hourglass as the ideal even though it only represents less than 1 in 10 of the female population. In the following pages we will show you how to get that perfect look but don't worry if you are off a little bit. The types above show that you'll still look like some females in the population and that means you'll fit right in as girl.

It's all in the proportions

A woman will often summarize herself by her vital statistics and compare herself to some 'ideal' numbers. These ideals are often criticised for not being realistic. We called our ideal Type 5 'Barbie' but the doll Barbie is quite controversial because her shape is not in proportion to what occurs naturally. Her hip to waist ratio is too low and her bust is far too big given her frame. Anyways, it is useful to have a guide bearing in mind that with a male frame you are not going to get these ideal numbers easily if at all. Understanding the idea of proportion though is crucial to getting a feminine look.

The classic shape is 36-26-36 measured in inches. Notice that the bust and hip sizes are the same, so this is like a rectangle squeezed in at the waist to make an hourglass. The ideal femme height is 5'8". That's on the taller end for women which tend to be about 5'5" tall or thereabout. So often you'll see women gaining the right height by wearing appropriate heels. If you do the maths, you'll see that the waist to hip ratio is 0.7. Obviously, women vary and so does the ratio. It can be as low as 0.65 and has high as 0.9. The number 0.8 is a good one to aim for. If you're heading to 0.9 you are more rectangle. If you are 0.65 that's tiny and on the sizes above would be a 'waspie' waist like you see in old movies with southern belles or Victorian dresses.

To be an hourglass the difference between the waist and hips or the waist and bust must be no less than 9". In the ideal measurements above you can see that this is 10" which meets the requirement. The bust must also be no-more than 2" bigger than the hips otherwise you're starting to look like Type 1. Vice-versa if the hips are more than 2" bigger than the bust then you're a cello or spoon shape and heading for a pear.

Let's do an example, if you are a 42-36-38 then your waist to hip ratio is 36/38 = 0.94 and differences for bust and hip are 42-36= 6" and 38-36=2" while the bust to hip difference is 42-38=4". Not quite the ideal. More like type 1. But if we could pull in your waist by 2" then your vitals would be 42-34-38 the numbers would be 34/38 = 0.89 and the differences 42-34=8", 38-34=4" and the bust to hip difference is still 4". Okay curvier but still a bit to do. Let's push out your hips by 2". Now your vitals are 42-34-40. You have a waist to hip ratio of 34/40 = 0.85 and differences of 42-34=8" and 40-34= 6" and the bust to hip difference is 42-40=2". Nearly there!

Let's push those hips out a bit more so your vitals are 42-34-42. Now the waist to hip ratio is 34/42 = 0.8, the differences are 42-34=8", and the hip to bust measurement is 42-42 = 0". See what we did? By adding 4" to your hips and taking 2" off your waist we got you almost hourglass. Of the three measures you are an inch under the 9" requirement. That's barely noticeable at any distance. All the others are good. Okay so you're not as petite as the ideal 36-26-36 (which are unrealistic anyway) but your feminine proportions are right. If people look at your silhouette they'll think girl.

The takeaway from all this maths is to use your own vital statistics and check the ratios and differences to see how close to hourglass you are. The most important point is that whatever your shape is we try and get it in proportion. Women do this in two ways. First is to get the overall body shape lined up so that it forms a sensuous sort of S-shape when you look front on or in three quarters position (slightly at an angle). This is the classic look that models use in fashion magazines. The second is to consider your bust and butt size so that from the front it is full and rounded but also in proportion on a side profile. We'll focus on your boobs in the next chapter and your butt in the chapter after that.

Changing your body type

What kind of reductions or increases are we talking about? Not huge – 2-4 inches maximum. If you pad out the hips 4 inches and pull in the waist 4 inches that is a difference of eight inches. That's a lot. But if you take the minimum change of 2" for each that is 4 inches difference in total. That's not bad at all. If you have a reasonable sized man hand the length of your thumb is about 2". Adding 1-2" (or a thumb's length) to both sides of your hips or taking it off your waist will do the trick. That's all! Most people can manage that.

As practice let's consider each type and see how we can create a pleasing shape. If we consider Type 1, then there can be two problems no hips and/or a waist bigger than the hips. What we want to do is add on some size to the hips and then pull in the waist. The first step might get us back to rectangle and then the second gets us to hourglass.

In Type 2 the problem is the waist. We want to pull in the waist to rectangle and then if possible further in to hourglass. Type 3 is already rectangle so that is just pulling in the waist and if we want adding a bit to the hips. That will possibly make us look a bit pear shaped but wider hips if not overdone can be sexy. You've heard the phrase 'good child-bearing hips'? If you get this right, you can look very earth-mother. Imagine wearing a thin loose dress carrying a babe on your hip.

Type 5 is the classy hourglass so already very feminine but check the proportions. How hourglass is it? Do the bust and hips line-up and how do they fit in relation to the overall numbers? Are you a cello or a spoon? You might want to add something to the hips to balance up. Alternatively, if you pull in the waist a touch you might look naturally more petite or voluptuous. Alternatively, you might think about adding some fullness to your bust as a distracter. The next chapter will show you how to get a designer bust and Part 3 will show you how downplay your wider shoulders with cuts of clothing and other embellishments.

Play with the numbers. Step 1 get yourself back to the rectangle shape by padding out the hips. There are lots of girl clothes you can wear as a rectangle and with the right walk and mannerisms you'll pass as female. Step 2 see to what degree you can pull in the waist to get something approximating the hourglass. Best to avoid too much pull in because it all must go somewhere and that is usually to press in on your internal organs. You want to be comfortable when you dress not trussed up like a turkey.

What about Type 4 (the pear)? No, we didn't forget about it, but it is a bit of a problem. Evidence of this is clear to see in women's magazines and fashion websites. The hips and the waist might be in the right proportion but the hips are too big (bigger than the shoulders). The only option is to make your shoulders or bust look wider. Not easy. We can give the illusion if you choose the right clothes or make you boobs fuller. We'll look at how cuts of clothes and patterns can disguise your underlying shape in Part 3 of the book. Skip there now if you want a sneak preview.

Shapewear

Okay, so no matter what shape you are there is something we can do to make you more feminine looking. Don't worry if your vitals aren't working for you. Women have all sorts of tricks to make it happen and the number one secret is shapewear.

The idea of using clothing or other aids to alter your shape goes back to ancient times. The first shape shifters were the Greeks who used a form of girdle to cinch the waist and push out the breasts. Roman women used corsets to enhance their curves and eventually wore them on the outside of clothing making them fashion accessories with embroidery and studs. Roman women would also strap their breasts to make them look smaller and rounder. In the 16th century steel corsets were introduced which kept the figure flat on the tummy and pulled in at the waist. Skirts were freer emphasizing the hips.

The Victorian era was when the hourglass first became the ideal model. Steel and whalebone corsets were used to pull virtually any figure into the classic shape. The compression on the body could be so great that women would often faint when excited or over exerted. In hot countries a lady would retire to her boudoir in the afternoon to loosen up. This all added to the view that women were the 'weaker' sex.

In the original *Pirates of the Caribbean* film there is a funny scene where Elizabeth, played by Kiera Knightly, is so tightly bound that she faints from all the excitement. But it is not so far from the truth. In days of old when women wore tight corsets, they faced all sorts of health issues from fainting to breathlessness and problems with their internal workings. That waspie 22" waist that Cinderella has, or you see in Disney films, is to die for, sometimes literally. Let's be sensible.

In the 20th century these extreme practises fell out of favour – not least because of the health problems but also because steel was needed for the war effort. Women were encouraged not to wear corsets. Between the first and second world wars women preferred the rectangle look with fitted shapers like teddies and camisoles. Dresses were flat and thin. Because of this flimsiness they were referred to as flappers. After the second world war and into the 1950s and 60s the girdle and corset had a revival but used more modern materials such as elastic which could be made into panels to act as control and shapers.

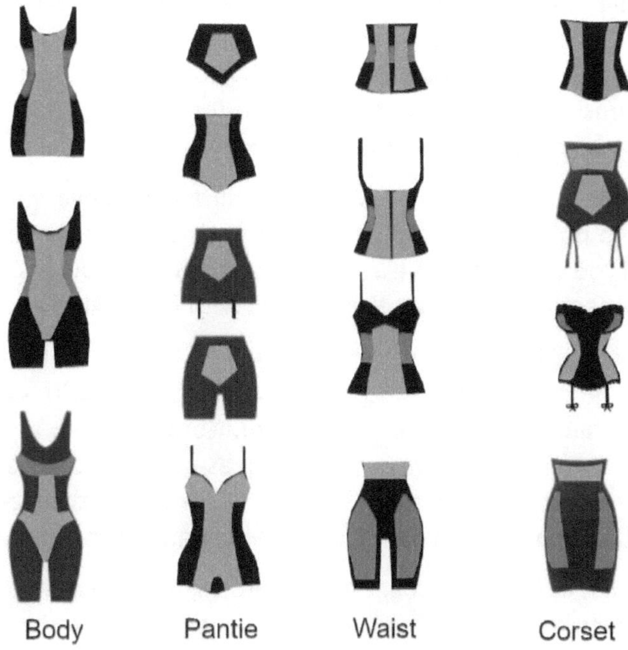

Figure 3 options for shapewear

Now we have all sorts of ways to control body shape. The elastic panel approach is the most popular and that is what we consider here. In the section on lingerie we will look at the more traditional corset which has a reputation for naughtiness and sensuality.

The collective name we give to shapewear are foundation garments. That is exactly what they do – create a foundation for your feminine appearance. Most women's clothes shops or on-line stores will have a section on foundation or control garments and there are some special forms especially for crossdressers which can be found in more specialist outlets. The materials are more advanced than in the past so that they can be lightweight, comfortable, and flexible to body movement.

Girdles

The main item of clothing we are looking for is a girdle. Girdles come in a variety of forms depending on what you need to achieve. Figure 3 shows the main types with the grey areas showing where the main control panel is positioned. The black areas will also be tighter than usual clothing to give a firm fit.

Body Girdle: this covers most of the torso (can include the boobs and thighs or not). It slims the waist and thigh areas but leaves the buttocks untouched. Because it covers the whole torso this one is good with figure hugging dresses like the modern bodycon (or body contour) look that is popular with young or businesswomen today.

Waist Girdle: this gridle fits under your bust and above your hips. It is designed to pull in your waist to give you the hourglass shape. This one is good if all you want is to have a narrow waist and use trouser or pants suits to avoid a pantie line but can also be used with fuller skirts and blouses.

Open Girdle: as its name suggests has an open bottom that extends down over the thighs and buttocks. Sometimes is can be used with suspenders or as a garter belt itself (see lingerie section). Normally it has a panel on the front that flattens the tummy area as well as pulling in the waist. A great choice for wider circle skirts, 50s style dresses and petticoats where the garters attachments are hidden but you also want a flat tummy.

Panty Girdle: as the name suggests this girdle is like a 'bigger' pair of pants. The fit can be anywhere from just under your waistline to just under your bust area and can also extend downwards with longer legs or have garters to use with stockings in an open style. Again, there is a panel in the front which is used to pull in the tummy and lower abdomen area to give a flat stomach and trim the midsection. This looks great with things like pencil skirts. A lot of crossdressers start with a panty girdle because it is what their mothers wore and if there is an extension over the top of the legs it hides your male bits quite effectively.

Vintage Girdles: are the old-style Victorian corsets that come in a variety of forms. They are usually very tight fitting. Sometimes they have clasps or laces so that you can pull the waist right in. Compared to the other types of girdle they are more fashionable and come in a variety of styles. You can of course wear them over the top of the other types of girdles for multiple areas of control or as a fashion accessory over a shirt or blouse.

Crossdressing Girdles: these types of girdles are specifically designed for male to female transformation. In addition to the styles above they also come with pockets built into the fabric. The pockets are used for padding. For example, hip, butt, or thigh pads. Placing the right size and shape pad into the pocket will bulk out your figure but also create a smooth line when you wear dresses or even tighter fitting skirts and outfits. This is the way to add size rather than pulling it in (see Figure 4 below).

Armed with your body type and vital statistics you need to decide what types of foundation wear you need. If you need only to pull in the waist use a vintage style corset. If you want to flatten the tummy go with a panty gridle with the options to add bottom pads. Use the longer girdles over the buttocks and thighs to add thigh padding. The more changes you need the more you'll need to move towards the full body girdle.

Think it over and decide what your options are. The best advice is to use the minimum padding to get the best look you can. That way you will have more flexibility in the clothes you can wear. It is a trade-off between how unencumbered you feel and how feminine you look. If you are happy with your figure don't use any control clothing at all. Most people though like to flatten or smooth out their figure to some degree.

Waist Training

Shapewear is a temporary fix. It sucks you in or pads you out as long as you are wearing it. If you are looking for something more permanent an alternative is to retrain your body posture.

Waist training is rather controversial because of its notoriety from Victoria times. Doctors will tell you that it does nothing to help you lose weight (or fat) which superficially is true and that the inward push will squeeze your organs pushing your lungs and heart together and squashing your intestines together with your lower organs. As a result, you may be short of breath or cause heart problems. Alternatively, block bowel movements creating constipation among other things. All of this is true if you go at it willy nilly and don't watch your health.

The counter view is that female anatomy, particularly, is used to the organs moving around because that is what happens in pregnancy as the womb grows. The same is true of the male when we exercise. The restriction of a corset will make your body work harder with any exercises generating more heat and sweat which will help you burn energy and fat. And, the restriction on the tummy area will confine the stomach so you will eat less.

Other people will say that waist training is a fantasy. Maybe because they tried it and it didn't work for them. If you wear a fashion or lingerie corset or the shapewear above, there is virtually zero chance that it will make a long-term difference to your waist profile. Waist training works a little bit like braces to straighten your teeth. It gradually adjusts the natural sit of your body over a long period of time. So you need to be dedicated if this is what you want.

To be effective you need to use a corset with steel or bone supports. These can be laced tight and push in your body. If you wear them regularly (like every day) then they will train your fatty tissues to take on a different shape that moulds more to the shape of the corset. And, the steel frame will be able to push in the bottom few (floating or false) ribs which are not attached to your sternum and depend more on cartilage for position. These two things will give a tapering from your upper ribs and hips in towards a slimmer waist as well as flattening your tummy area. The tightness of the corset will also give you a more upright posture by straightening your back. Altogether this will make you look more hourglass.

If waist training appeals then here are a few tips on getting started:

Get the right sized corset: so that you can pull it in over a period of time. Going too small too quickly will create all sorts of problems and it won't get you there faster. Corsets come in two sizing ranges – standard and plus sizes. Sizes under 32 are considered standard and 34-46 are plus sized.

Choose a corset style that fits your body type. For this we are interested in the length of your torso. The torso is measured from just under your bust to the top of your legs. Do this by sitting down, sitting up straight, and measuring the vertical. You are standard size if the length is 8". Long is about 11" and short is 7.5" or less. If you are long, you will need to consider a longline corset. If you are short, then a waspie will do the trick. Waspies also work for the other sizes too but really pull in which might not be what you need initially.

Choose the shape and curve: a waspie has an extreme curve and is short so suited to hippy people with short torsos. Best to avoid if you are already hourglass or have a bit of muffin top going on. The standard corset has a minimal curve and suits the more athletic looking person with some curves. Use a hybrid corset (with bust) that fits higher on the back if you have a longer torso and can take a smoother curve in to the waist. Long corsets will suit most body types and can have varying degrees of curve. It all depends on what sort of shape you are aiming for as your final goal.

Choose your material: corsets come in all sort of materials (see lingerie section) since you will be wearing it a lot you want comfort, breathability and durability. The best choice is cotton, but you may decide to have more than one corset of different styles. You should always wear a liner between your skin and the corset. The natural oils in your skin or your moisturisers and skin care products can soak in or affect the material, so this keeps them clean and fresh. Note that most corsets need dry cleaning so look after them if you want to avoid too many trips to a cleaner and moments of embarrassment.

Season your corset: don't tighten your corset as far as you can the first few times you wear it. Also, you need to loosen up the lace holes and so on. Ideally, the first few times you should be able to easily slip your flat hand into the top and bottom. You may also find that the modesty panel (the rectangle of fabric behind the laces) doesn't quite join up. Obviously, some of this depends on your measurements and how much material you are squashing in. The corset has to be broken in otherwise you will warp the steel or boning and making it painful to wear.

Limit you first time use: wear your corset only about 1-2 hours the first time. Repeat this several times over the next few days so that the material slowly stretches to a comfortable fit. This is also good advice if you are using a fashion corset or intend to wear one only for a special occasion. This way you will feel comfortable and also gain sexy curves.

Tighten up gradually: when you put on the corset lace it up slowly so that you get a nice snug fit. Go in a series of stages to your preferred tightness. Don't ever tighten to the point where it is painful or hard to breathe. Start wearing your corset for 1-2 hrs a day and then build that up to 6-8 hours. You should do this over about two weeks. Once you get up to a significant time start to pull in the corset more and more over the coming weeks. This will give time for your body to adjust. You should start to notice some changes after about 4 weeks but it can take years to get a tiny waist.

Take breaks: initially you'll find that some days you can wear the corset for longer and other days it feels impossible. Don't beat yourself up and take a few days break every now and then. If you feel pain, are breathless, or any part of you feels numb then the corset is too tight. Take a break and when you restart don't tighten up as much. Only go at the pace that your body indicates is okay.

To keep things healthy, it is a good idea to watch your diet to help slim even further and to exercise to tone up the core muscles and fascia for better posture. Never do heavy exercise in your corset this will only cause you breathing difficulties and restrict your body's ability to stretch when it needs to. Some people also like to continue their training while they are asleep. In these cases, loosen your corset so that it is 1-2" more flexible than during the daytime. This will allow your body to relax and recover. You will also sleep better.

The final results depend on your anatomy and the degree to which you can stick at it. Don't rush. Just for information the world record is a 15" waist (aka Cathie Jung) achieved after many years of training. Ethel Granger is supposed to have had the smallest ever waist at 13". The type of figure you see in Disney films or Princess dresses is at about 22". In the book - *Gone with the wind* – the main character Scarlett boasts of a 17" waist but Vivien Leigh who played her in the famous film was 25" in her dress. Vivien was also on the smaller side of female frame at 5'3" tall. The ideal woman size is just over 26". But the average real woman today is about 36". Use these numbers to set realistic expectations for yourself.

Waist training can turn into a bit of an obsession. Please be sensible and remember you're starting out with more of a waist than these female examples. A natural waist circumference of more than 35" in women and 40" in men puts you at a higher risk of disease. A large waist indicates that you have a lot of visceral fat. That's the type of fact that is around your organs not the subcutaneous fat just under the skin. This deeper fat is a higher risk factor for breast cancer, gallbladder issues, heart disease, and diabetes. If this applies to you then it means waist training is a higher risk activity. Any compression could be dangerous. If you have any worries or concerns check yourself out with a doctor before you start any training.

DIY padding

Padding fills you out rather than pulling you in. If you find that pads are too expensive, or you don't like the fit, consider making your own. One reason for this approach is that shapewear pads unless from a crossdressing store might be on the thin side compared to the size of extension you need. This is because they are designed for women who already have a lower hip to waist ratio and some thigh/buttock fat. Likewise, the cheaper pads can move more or give you some lines through your clothing. Fitting to your own shape is the ideal solution.

Making a pair of pads is not rocket science. There are three stages required. First is getting a shape to make a template from. Second is finding a suitable material. And, third is cutting to shape for a smooth finish. By far the most accessible, cost effective and easiest material to get hold of is foam used for furniture manufacture. Get the high-density version because otherwise the pad will press in too much when your clothing is tight. This can be bought in strips or rolls. You'll need something in the region of

100cm (1 yard) by 75 cm (2 feet) and at least 5cm (or 2 inches) of thickness for each pad. A square seat cushion is just about the right size and has enough thickness for you to trim back to a decent finish.

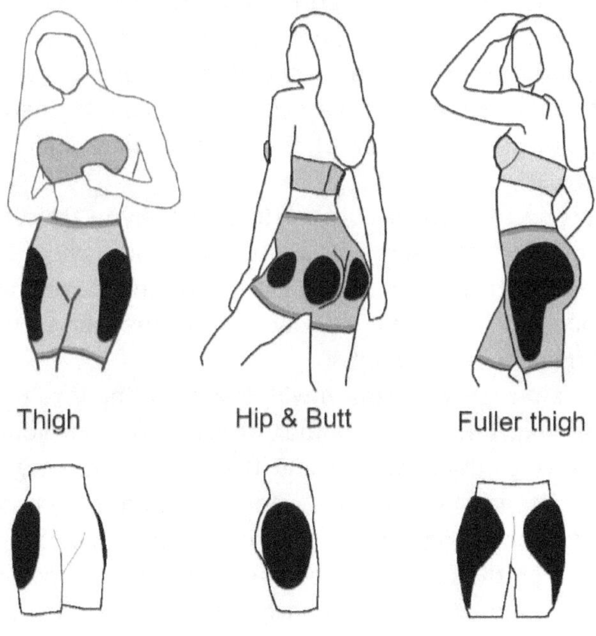

Figure 4 Padding for extra curviness

Look at the pads in Figure 4 and decide which ones you want to make. You'll need three measurements. First is the vertical length down the leg from just where the hip forms from the waist to where the major muscle ends above your knee or higher depending on what length you want or the clothes you are planning to wear. Second find the measurement around the top of your leg and as far into the butt area that you want to go. Third measure the width around the outside of the lower thigh for the narrowest area of the pad.

Get a piece of card (or paper) and transfer these horizontal and vertical measurements, marking off the top, bottom and sides. Sketch out the outline of the pad from figure 4 that you want. It doesn't have to be a work of art. No one is going to see it under your clothes just round off the curves, so it isn't too angular. Cut out the card to make the template. Next place the template on the foam and trace around the edge with a maker pen. Cut out the shape from the foam. You'll need two of these one for each leg, thigh, or butt cheek depending on the pad.

Now comes the most difficult bit. We need to sculpt the remaining foam so that it has a nice smooth rise towards the middle. Mark the place where your upper thigh will be widest with a cross and then make a small oval around the cross to define the area of maximum extension. Now we need to taper the edges of the pad up to this point. There are a variety of ways to do this using a pair of scissors or a sharp knife. Obviously watch your fingers!!

It is better if you secure the foam while you are cutting. Start at the edges and take small slices off as you work your way to the central raised area. This can take some time. Take it slow and make it as smooth as you can. While you are shaping think about how the pad will wrap around your leg and the curves you want.

An alternative approach with less sculpting is to use something like yoga matting. Cut out a number of sections from your template each slightly smaller than the last and then stack them together to make a smooth flattened pyramid shape for the extension you need. Make sure you have some strong bonding glue to stick the levels together securely and then just trim the edges between layers to get a smoother finish. Two to three layers should give you an inch or more of padding.

Once you have finished the first pad hold it up to body to test the fit and adjust. Remember you need to stay in proportion so keep the extension no more than necessary to bring your hips out to somewhere between your chest and shoulders. Don't go beyond the shoulders otherwise you'll be a pear. When you are satisfied repeat the process for the second pad but use the first one as a visual guide while you are sculpting. Remember one is left and the other is right.

When you are finished pop them both inside your foundation garment or an elasticated body stocking. Now dress as desired and check out your curves. Just wearing the pads might feel a little John Wayne at first – like you are a gun fighter toting sidearms. But once you are dressed, you'll see that they make you look girly and curvy.

Of course, the downside of padding is that you're not going to be ripping your clothes off in a fit of passion. So more useful if you are dressing socially. That said, the so-called directoire style with silky pants, camisoles and slips over shapewear has some erotic allure especially in clothed female nude male (cfnm) scenarios. If you have a mistress or someone who is feminizing you, you might find that they get their sleek look from using control wear. If you are more mature in years then this can also be an attractive female look especially with 1950s and 60s attire where skirts, petticoats, stockings and tight bodice dresses were the in thing.

Shopping list

Don't just buy the first thing you find just to get the embarrassment over with. You only need one or two things depending on your type which is summarized below. Ask about the breathability, comfort, and durability. This piece of clothing is going under all your other femme clothes so you're going to want air to get in an out so you don't expire with heat or sweat (or should that be perspire – ladies say perspire.)

Type 1 (strawberry):

What you have: Wide shoulders, Narrow hips, flat bottom. *What you need:* Side hip extension, fattening of the bottom: *Shapewear required:* Panty girdle to lift bottom with cheek pads and or thigh padding.

Type 2 (apple):

What you have: Fuller waist. *What you need:* Defined waist. *Shapewear required:* Waist girdle.

Type 3 (banana): *What you have:* Little or no waist definition. Bottom may also be a little flat. *What you need:* Defined waist, lifting of the bottom. *Shapewear required:* Panty girdle with high waist. Pads to fill out and raise bottom. Control panels to flatten tummy and pull in waist.

Type 4 (pear): *What you have:* Full hips and thighs, Narrow shoulders. *What you need:* Tight control on the hips and thighs to pull them in. Firming of the bottom. *Shapewear required:* Extended or open girdle to add definition to lower torso

Type 5 (hourglass): *What you have:* Clearly defined waist. *What you need:* Balanced hip and bust, overall toning with a little pull in on the waist. Trim thighs and Flatter tummy. *Shapewear required:* Full girdle to tighten figure overall with control panels to bring in tummy.

Next is comfort, you don't want the thing ruching up, chafing or causing unsightly wrinkles or bulges. Although the control parts are often made of panels the rest of the garment will be tighter than usual clothing. The rest of the material should ideally be a type of cotton weave so that it is soft on the skin. You are going to be wearing these items of clothing a lot so you want to make sure that they are designed to last and can stand up to regular cleaning. Anything else is a false economy.

Shapewear items tend to be a bit more expensive than ordinary under things. Control pants and cinchers enter at about 10-20 dollars/pounds for a reasonable quality item. Items with control panels, some padding for thighs and pants for butt lifts come in at 30 upwards. A full body suit 20-30. Specialist crossdressing sites are a little more expensive because the parts are designed for the male anatomy and have a smaller market. Butt, thigh, hip and other shaper pads can be 40-50 upwards and full upper leg pads even more. If this is too much for you consider the DIY route.

If you don't need (or want) padding buy the regular girdles available in women's stores. Although male enquiries are not the norm modern customer service training means they will deal with you professionally. If you know your sizes and what you want order discreetly on-line.

And finally ...

The vital statistics (when wearing your shapewear), height and weight help to determine your dress and clothes sizes. You will need all these numbers if things are going to fit properly. Sometimes the width of your shoulders and length from your neck to your butt crease will also help determine a good fit.

Since a lot of female clothing is tailored if your back and shoulders are larger for your height than the female equivalent, you'll get an imperfect fit. Likewise, with the curve of a dress over your butt. The female pelvis is wider and tipped backward which gives a rounder bottom shape which makes a difference in fitted dresses or skirts. And, for fitted bodices your floating ribs won't taper in like the hourglass so that will pull the material in the back which might be hard or impossible to zip up even if they are your size. If things are going to be tight or close cut and the material is not stretchy go up a size.

Some manufacturers label clothes by the body types we have looked at above. But even though you are in proportion unless you are in the female height range (5'4"- 5'6") then you'll be better looking for the plus-sizes. Unless you are naturally woman sized you just won't get the fit you require because of the above differences in anatomy. This means you need to look at plus-size stores for some of your clothing. There are specialist stores that sell only plus size women clothing and lingerie so that is the best place to start. And, of course, crossdressing outlets or on-line shops will be sympathetic and understand what your needs are. Just search with the keywords: foundation wear, shape wear, plus size, and/or crossdressing and you'll find a whole list of stores or web places for your region.

Measuring for women's clothes is much more diverse than for men. Most international retailers use a small, standard, or large category but these ranges vary widely. Always check the retailers chart to convert your vitals to the right size. If you cannot find your sizes on the sizing chart it means you are either petite (smaller than average) or lean/tall (larger than the average) or curvy (wider than the average).

As a guide look at the table below which shows UK women's sizes. You can get US sizes by subtracting 4. The famous size zero dress that made all the news a few years ago is actually a size 4 in the UK. Plus size is generally considered to be anything above 18 (up to 32) but many stores start their bigger sizes at 14. The advantage of a crossdressing store is that they will stock the bigger sizes that fit men or have them specially made. But the downside is it is a specialist shop so the prices will go up. Buy from women's shops if you can – its also more girly and fun if you can just walk-in off the street and buy something.

UK size	Bust (inch/cms)	Waist (inch/cms)	Hips (inch/cms)
4	31 (78)	24 (60)	33 (83.5)
6	32 (80.5)	25 (62.5)	34 (86)
8	33 (83)	26 (65)	35 (98.5)
10	35 (88)	28 (70)	37 (93.5)
12	37 (93)	30 (75)	39 (98.5)
14	39 (98)	31 (80)	41 (103.5)
16	41 (103)	33 (85)	43 (108.5)
18	44 (110.5)	36 (92.5)	46 (116)

Finally, a word on vanity sizing. If your look is retro or vintage and you hunt online for authentic dresses be aware that as time has gone on sizes have gotten smaller. For example, a size 12 in the 1950s is a size 6 today. This is partly to do with the modern-day obsession with smaller sizes. Manufacturers have changed the numbers so people think they are skinny even though dresses are bigger sizes.

Another reason is because there are now a wider range of sizes available. In the past a lot of clothes were made from sewing patterns not bought off the peg. Anyway, make sure you check your numbers before you buy and end up with something that doesn't fit. It makes sense to ask the person you are buying from what the modern-day equivalent size is or just give your vital statistics and ask if it will fit.

If all else fails and you can hold a needle buy a dress pattern and some material and make your own. That way you can pin it and size it as you go. If your look is more retro there are lots of clothes patterns on-line and many of the classic catalogue ones are now collectibles. There are many many adorable nightwear patterns to make up which you just cannot buy in shops anymore and suit the crossdresser. Sissy clothes makers will make you something to order if you know what you want.

Chapter 5 The perfect Bust

Having got your curves right from the front it is now time to consider your side profile. It may sound crude but really most guys are first attracted by tits or tush. Brain experiments show that when a man is shown pictures of attractive women their eyes instinctively check out these bits and light up visualization centres as though they are checking against some universal standard of desirability. Even another woman will discreetly check these bits of anatomy to see if you are a rival. And, guess what, if what you have is ample or modest as long as it is all in proportion with the rest of your curves you will be attractive to a wide range of people.

The size, shape and weight of your bust will affect your centre of gravity and so influence how you hold and carry yourself, how you sit, and the type of clothes you can wear. It is not just a matter of stuffing your bra with something from the sock draw to give you a bit of frontage. In the following pages we'll look at breast anatomy and how that influences bra sizes and the type of bras you can buy to give this most important area a lift or create an appealing cleavage. If you're not interested in any of this and just want some bumps in your jumper, we will show you how to get the right weight and size that's right for your body type. The choices you make for your boobs can make the difference between being sensual, slutty, cute or demure.

What you need in the chest area depends on what you already have. Either you are flat chested (including developed pecs), have some man-boob thing going on, have implants already or are developing breasts as part of your transition. If you are the former, great we can design whatever you want size wise. If you are carrying some fat or breast tissue, there are ways we can exploit that to create a natural looking bust. It may be small and endearing as opposed to deep and voluptuous but hey it is you!

If you are in transition, have implants, or both you are developing like any girl so all you really need to do is learn how to buy the right bra.

That can be trickier than you imagine. You might want to pad a little like young women do until you fully develop or to give you more fullness. We'll show you how to do all that.

Breast Sizes and Weight

There are lots of euphemisms for your fun bags but they all imply something about the shape, weight, or symmetry. Girls tend to be demure on this referring to them as puppies, twins, the girls, boobs (or boobies), seeing them as a pair. Whereas men are more graphic as in jugs, melons, honkers, bristols, tits and a load of other crudities. Love them or hate them each reference conjures up a picture of size, weight and look. So, how do we formally classify boobs?

Women are interested in lots of things not just the size or roundness. For example, how even the two are, how symmetrical they are on your chest, whether they sag downwards, are perky, or fall to the side. Nipple size and position is also important. And despite what you might think boobs never point upwards even if that is how pinup girls are portrayed. It's all about gravity. Which eventually wins out. As a woman ages her boobs sag and fall sideways. An important function of a bra therefore is to support the weight and round those puppies up so they look perfect and perky. If you look too pert for your age though or too big for your frame, you'll draw attention to your dressing.

A busty girl has a fullness and deeper cleavage. Your bust doesn't have to be huge but if it is on the larger size compared to your body frame, you'll be more voluptuous and milk maid. Another thing is good size nipples. This includes areola (or the dark patches around the nipple itself) as well as stiffness. A glimpse or hint of nipple under your clothing will excite and tease. If you think that is slutty and cheap then it is easy to choose garments that keep things gentle and more circumspect.

Anyways what can we say about the size and shape of breasts compared to your frame. Typically, breasts are tear-dropped shaped not balloon shaped. A fuller breast appears rounder and fuller but doesn't lose the tear drop shape (see Figure 5). The tissue hangs off the chest with the weight centred at the lower end. A useful way to think of this is as saddlebags around your neck. When you put on your bra any breast form you use will have to be supported by your neck and upper torso.

A bra is cleverly designed to help support the weight. The number one rookie mistake in giving yourself a pair of boobs is to make them too round or big. If you want your boobs to look realistic and move in the right way when you bend or stretch, you'll have to think about how the weight pulls the breast into that teardrop shape and hangs off the chest.

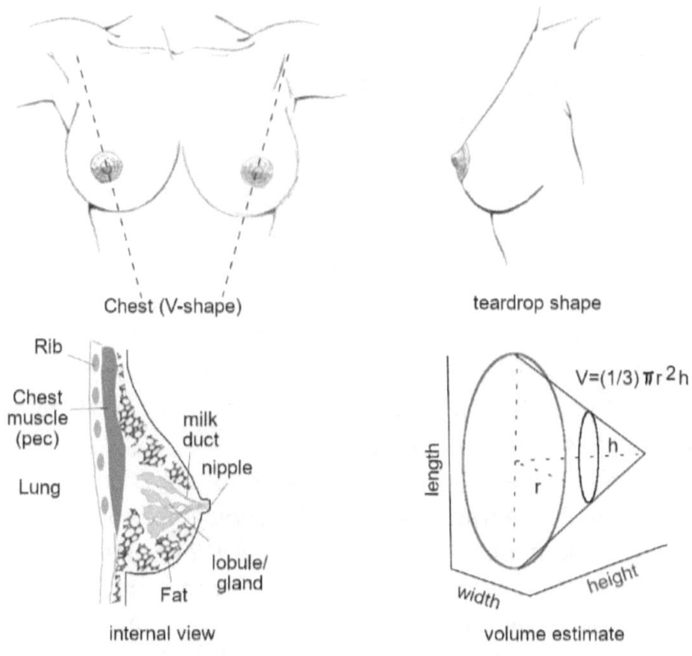

Figure 5 Breast structure and size

So how much do boobs actually weigh? To calculate the weight, we need to figure out the volume of breast material. Suppose for simplicity that we imagine a breast as a circular cone shape (think Madonna in that Vogue video). If you remember your high school maths the volume can be given by the formula $V = (1/3) \pi r^2 h$. Boob volume depends on the size of the circle on your chest (r = radius of the circle) and the distance it projects off your chest (h = height). Since you have two even sized breasts the radius is about a quarter of the width of your chest. The height can be found by measuring around the boobs and then subtracting it from the band size (that is the distance around the bottom of your ribcage). Just to confuse things when you buy bras and other stuff the cup size is given a letter. An 'A' is roughly equivalent to a height of 1", a B is 2", a C is 3" and so on from which the volume and size of cup can be estimated.

Now we can add that to your vital statistics. The fashion industries ideal woman has the bust-waist-hip measurements 36C-26-36. The letter tells you the size of her breasts. She has a projection of her bust approximately 3" out from her chest. And chest width is going to be something like 10" given that the bust measurement goes around the torso. That is about half the total (18) minus a bit for the sides (8). As each breast covers half the chest the diameter of the circle is 5" and the radius (r) is about 2". Stick the numbers in the formula and you have the volume. It is about 37.68 cubic inches.

Now we have to convert that to a weight. A cubic inch of water weighs 0.036 pounds. And it just so happens that boob flesh is about 0.9 the weight of water. Don't ask me why. It's a magic number. Or perhaps has something to do with the fact that human cells are mostly fluid. Anyways. We can work out the ideal girl breast weight as 37.68 x 0.036 = 1.36 pounds of water and convert that to flesh by 0.9 x 1.36 = 1.22 pounds. That is one breast so the actual weight she is carrying on her chest is double that or 2.44 pounds. If you want it in metric, 1g = 0.0022 lbs so that is an estimate of 554 grams per breast.

To find the weight of your own boobs or man boobs you can do it by displacement. Find a tray and a bowl big enough for you to dip your breast tissue into without touching bottom or sides. Weigh the tray and record the measurement. Fill the bowl up to the rim with warm water. The warm water is for your comfort. Now stick all your boob into the water so that it is kind of floating and let it settle. Water will spill out onto the tray. Now take the bowl off the tray and measure the weight of the tray and water combined. Subtract the weight of the tray. Now you have the weight of the water equivalent to the volume of your boob. To convert it into a breast weight just multiply by the magic number 0.9.

If you think you don't have anything to work with. Trust me, unless you are super fit or skinny-as-a-rake you probably have a little A-cup or a small B with the fat on your chest. We'll show you how to use all this to find the ideal breasts so just play along for the moment and learn what all the letters and numbers mean. You're going to need them to buy bras or clothes or order things like breast forms and padding so it is well worth the effort.

Bra and Bust sizes

A bra is designed to help support the breast weight and it does this by comprising three elements: the band, the cup, and the straps. The band goes around your ribcage under your breasts. The cup holds the flesh of the breast. The shoulder straps help support the weight and join the cup to the band. Together the ensemble can be adjusted to help lift, round, and push the breasts into a pleasing feminine shape. When boobs look terrible it is because the bra doesn't fit properly or is not adjusted correctly. A bra is classified by a band size and a cup size. The band is a number and the cup size a letter. The average woman is a 36C/D.

The first thing to note is that the bigger the boobs the heavier they are going to be. Most men think of breasts like little squidgy balloons. If you are going to dress regularly you need proper support to carry any weight on your chest. Too much weight and long term they will hurt your back and pull your shoulders and spine down. Big breasted women often opt for breast reduction surgery when they get older to help with posture and back pain.

What size bra do you need? This sounds like a simple question, but it isn't. Bra manufacturers have a funny way of classifying bras which is based on our boob weighing experiments in the previous section. Suppose you measure your vital statistics and come out as a 39B. Simple right? You look in the store for the bra with the label 39B. Except you won't find one. Bra sizes only come with even sized band numbers. If you were a 39 (or any odd number) then you'd have to round up or down to choose a bra either taking a 38 or a 40. Basically, if you tried the 38 and it was tight, you'd go up to 40. If a 40 was loose and shifting up your back, you'd go down to a 38.

Bras have catches on the back of the band so you can easily adjust an inch or so to get a nice fit. But you'd still have to have the right volume in the cups for it to fit properly. The bra straps have sliders on them so you can pull the cup up to get a tighter fit and lift the breast to make it more perky but if there is more material than breast volume that's not going to work very well. And if you don't have enough material for the volume you're going to be popping out when you move. Often busty looking girls aren't that big-breasted their bras are just tight.

So, here's the question –do 38B, 39B and 40B all have the same cup size? You'd think so but that is not true. To cut a long story short the boffins in the bra design lab measured lots of women and came up with a method called sister sizing. Sister sizing uses the fact that the volume of a breast is related to the size of your body. Bigger people, on average, tend to have bigger breasts. Smaller people, on the whole, have smaller breasts. They use this information to create a 'true' cup size for people with different band sizes and then make variations for the other breast sizes. A true A-cup breast weighs 236.3g, B-cups 447.5g and C-cups 531.5 g. Remember our calculations in the last section.

Take two women (sisters say) of different height and frame. Their boobs will look proportionally bigger or smaller when compared to the size of the rest of the body. What the boffins realised was that if you have, say, a band of size 36 then your breast size (the difference between bust and chest measures) is probably going to be about 3" (or a C). That is 36C is the true bra and cup size for that type of person. Likewise suppose your sister has a band size of 34 then she probably, on average, has a bust to chest size of 2" (or a 34B), another true cup-size. This is all based on statistics, so the true size represents the breast size of an average woman of a given height and frame as measured by the band size. In reality boobs may be smaller or bigger than this because we are all different even if we have the same band measurement.

Now for the tricky bit. Let's compare sisters again. Suppose that they both get a chest-bust-band measurement of 2" do they have the same breast volume? Not really. Think of our simplified breast as the circular cone shape in Figure 5. The circle is on the flat of your chest and the cone sticks outward coming to a point at the nipple. The height of the cone is 2" for both sisters. But boobs always fit fully across the chest. The size 34 sister has smaller circles than the size 36 sister for the same projection. Hence, their volumes are different for the same measurement because although height (h) is the same the radius (r) is different. Size B does not mean the same thing for the two sisters. Bras 34B and 36B do not have the same cup size. A 36B needs more material in the cup to hold the volume than in a 34B.

Here is how sister sizing works. You measure yourself and get an odd number for the bust size and a 2" difference between band and bust. If you got 39 you have to choose a 38 or a 40 bra. But which cup size? What does your chest-bust number of 2" mean? The boffins used the above argument to link cup volume and band size. Only a 32A is a true A-cup (as we measured it). Likewise, a 34B is the only true B-cup. And a 36C the only true C cup. The cup volume of a 40A is the same as a 38B, which is the same as a 36C or a 34D. Can you see the pattern? As the numbers go down the letter goes up.

Now you can choose your correct bra. If you measured at 39B then try a 40B and if the band is too loose go to the next size down 38C (not B). Alternatively, try the 38B and if that is too tight on the band go up to 40A (not B). Likewise, if you are not a true size, that is you're not a 32A, 34B, 36C etc. you can look at your sister sizes to get a better fitting cup. Example, you are a 34C which is not a true C-cup, then you could try a 32D or a 36B.

Use the catches on the bra to compensate for the change in band and the sliders to fit the cup.

Why is all this so complicated? Well manufacturers want to make only a limited range of bras that fit the most people. It's all about economics. Once you understand this, sizing is easy. It's also worth noting that 'Barbie' sizes like DD, FF, an GG are also just amendments to the scale of lettering. For example, most women will fit in the A-D range. What happens if you are an E, F, or G. That's simple the scale stops a D and we just keep adding the same letter. So 32E is 32DD and 30F is 30DDD. So double D doesn't mean you are twice as big as a D. It means the next size up from D. That is an extra inch on the projection out from the chest but that can add quite a lot of volume.

Think of the cones and formula. Do the maths for FF (size F plus one) and GG (size G plus 1) and you'll see that these are still quite substantial sizes. Very large breasts can run to 3, 4, or 5 thousand grams. That's over six times bigger than the average C. These kinds of bigger breasts might be popular with showgirls or drag queens but not for a passable look. And, do your really want to be lugging all that weight around. For a passable look try and stick in the A-D range.

Now you might think we are labouring all this a bit. Here are a few reasons why this knowledge is useful. First, the chances are that your current or new bra(s) won't fit you forever. You might gain weight and change your band size but not your breast size (especially if they a false ones). You will need to change your cup size to stay in proportion. Your band might stay the same and the breast might get bigger (e.g. as your transition continues or if you put on weight and deposit more fat on your chest). You might also want a couple of different sized bras to take account of manufacturer differences. For example, skimpy lingerie and play bras are often smaller than you think or come in one size only.

Staying in proportion (*V-shape and Y-shape*)

What does sister sizing mean for your feminization? Well we can use it as a method to choose our ideal breast size so that our body stays in proportion with our bust. No good having tiny boobs on a big body or for that matter big boobs on a tiny body. The average size for a woman is 36C (a true cup size).

One way to determine your ideal breast size is to use the true sizes to get to the closest for your actual frame. Find your bust measurement. If it is an odd number go up or down to get a band size (an even number).

Better to go down if you are bigger framed and are at the higher end of the scale. Now look at the scale 32A, 34B, 36C, 38D, 40E, 42F and so on. These are all true cup sizes. Find your band size and look at the letter. Remember the band is under your pecs (or breasts) and the bust around the chest. Now the conversion for the bust minus band is A=1", B=2" and so on. This is the projection of your boobs out from your chest. Suppose your band size is 40. That is an E (or DD) so your expected girl size or breast cone height is 5".

Get a tape measure and place one end on your breastbone in the middle of your chest between the boobs level with the nipples. Pull the tape out to the measured length this is the forward projection of your boobs. It is where your nipples would be on the curve of your breast. What do you think? Stand sideways and look at yourself in a mirror. Remember breasts are not balloons they are shaped more like flattened teardrops with the weight at the bottom. They should fall away from your chest gradually. If they look too big back off the measurement until you are happy. If they look too small extend a little but not too much. When you are satisfied take the reading on the tape measure and covert it back to a letter. The band number and letter are your breast or bust size. Add this to your vital statistics and you have a snapshot of your figure.

Another thing to look at is how your boobs match your other curves. Do they work together or does one look out of place? Are you top heavy? Dress sizes and lingerie are all cut to common sizes for women (even the plus sizes) so if you are buying stuff and its regularly not fitting it's a good sign that your curves and boobs are not in proportion. If your measurements are making you bigger then try and stay close to the average size for women (36C) or one of the sister sizes. Have a look at actresses and celebrities and check their vitals. Compare your own vital statistics and see how close to feminine you already are.

Don't get carried away with pushing up and inwards even if your cleavage is smaller or more open. The best look is a rounded Y for your chest but that only works if the breasts are fuller on the outside. As your cup size goes up the breasts have greater volume. The tear drop shape will swell so that they are more bell shaped. This adds fullness to the bottom of the breast. On the inside you get a better cleavage as the breast fills the gap between your boobs. And also rounds the outside so the boobs will extend out beyond the side of your torso. This can help balance your bottom half to get that hourglass look but also look barbie or bimbo if they are too wide.

To stay in proportion your nipple position must lie on a V between the shoulders (end of collar bones) and your crotch. This V shape is like a chevron pointing at your girl bits. The end of the shoulders are outside and the tummy button inside the V. Ideally, the boobs need to straddle the line as it tapers inwards. If the outside side of your boobs are inside this line, they will look squashed and lack fullness on the sides and are obviously fake. If they go too far outside this line they will look, loose, saggy and less perky. It won't look like you have any support. Try adjusting your bra so that the nipple position is on the line of the V and see what works best for you.

Filling the Cups

If you don't have any breast material, we will need to fill the cups. There are a variety of ways to do this depending on what you want to do while en-femme. For example, do you want to wear revealing dresses, do sports, wear swimsuits or loose clothes, dress occasionally or all the time, or sleep with your breasts in place. We'll look at three variations to accommodate these things: breast forms, padding, and au natural. As we move from one to the other there are a few things to keep in mind: weight, pliability, durability, quality, cost, and of course look. Dolly Parton famously said, 'it costs a lot of money to look this cheap.' She was being funny of course because she has a small frame and a big chest. But the reality is that it can cost you to look good.

Breast forms are clever inventions and get more sophisticated as technology in plastics, silicone, and moulding advance. Basically, a breast form is a moulding of a single breast. Originally, they were developed for women who lost their breasts due to mastectomy or had a deformation but have now been embraced by the crossdressing and trans community. Usually a woman will have a prosthetic designed specifically for her breast issue but there are now lots of off-the-shelf solutions. Crossdressing breasts have been designed with the male chest in mind.

The idea is simple you pop a couple into your bra and you're done. That's great but there are a few things to think about. First is that you obviously need two, one for each boob. But boobs are like feet you have a left one and a right one and the form of the left is the mirror of the right in terms of fullness on the outside edge. Make sure you have left and right in the correct cup – no banana boobs.

A breast form can come in different shapes but the most life-like are ones with that tear-drop shape. Some may have a nipple. Some are rounder or more pert than others. Breast forms usually come as flesh coloured but not always. Check for the right skin tone for you. Depending on the material they can be soft and pliable with some of the silicone ones most flesh like. If your breast form only comes in one shape (no left or right), then it probably rounder or more bell shaped. That's fine but you might not have any fullness at the sides which can make you look less curvy and full. To get that fullness you might need a bigger form than your measured cup size.

Good breast forms weigh the same as natural breasts of the same size, but some are very light or can be heavier depending on the material. This will affect your movement and how you carry your bust especially when bending over. The back surface of a form is smooth and/or contoured so that it can fit snugly against your chest or any breast material you already have. The back can also be made of material that holds well with adhesive. This means that with a smooth-shaven chest you can stick them on. This way they feel more realistic and part of you but importantly won't shuffle about or swing in the bra when you move.

Of course, you get what you pay for. Depending on budget you might have to compromise on the shaping of the breasts, the detail, finish and so on. Cheaper alternatives (tens of dollars) are foam which is sculptured into a breast shape but doesn't have the weight. The more expensive ones can be a few hundred dollars. An alternative is to buy a breast bra (or harness). This has a pair of breast forms connected to strapping like a bra but thinner. The idea is that your put them on and then a pretty bra over the top. A specially made crossdressing bra will have pockets in the cups that you can put your breast forms in to keep them secure. And sometimes the whole bra comes with the cups already filled. This is a choice if you are worried about the forms moving or dislodging. If your bra fits properly that shouldn't be a problem. Using ordinary bras is half the fun of dressing and will widen your fashion choices. Depends what you want.

Sometimes the way you move or how you sit can open up gaps between your clothing and your skin. This also applies to breast forms because they rest against the skin and it is difficult to hide the join. Hence you are confined to modest dress cuts with higher necklines or blouses and less revealing tops. Oh, and be aware, guys are going to look down your chest. They can't help it – honestly.

If you are sitting and they are standing this gives them the optimal view and if your clothing is too revealing they'll see your secret. Stick on breasts might seem a great idea and can be more discreet but if you are doing this regularly, you'll have to think about hygiene and keeping your own chest tissue healthy. Constantly applying and removing adhesive can make you sore. Another answer is a shapewear or full bra but that can look at bit matronly. Alternatively, but expensive (over 500 pounds/dollars) are halter style silicone tops. They cover all your chest and have the breasts built in.

Another thing to watch out for is flimsiness or transparency of clothing. If there is no nipple detail your boobs can look excessively smooth. Some people like that contoured look especially in tight dresses and T-shirts. If you do have the ones with nipple definition when you stretch or move the material of your dress or blouse may catch as it shifts across your boobs. That can look ultra-feminine. Also, if your breast forms are skin toned you can wear more girly or lingerie style bras and the tone will show through. Seeing the hint of flesh through your blouse or top material is also very sensual provided it is not too obvious and of course matches your own skin tone. Anything that adds to the mystique is good. But if you don't want any of that just go with the standard (cheaper) shape forming style inserts.

DIY breast forms

Every crossdresser at some point has improvised a breast form or two even if it is just stuffing socks in your bra. By the way that often comes out lumpy. The main problem with improvising is that your form won't necessarily keep the shape of a breast when pressed and it won't have the right weight. Nevertheless, if you are on a budget or don't want to buy breast forms what can you do.

The easiest approach is to take some appropriate fabric that won't easily burst or leak and fill it with appropriate material. Some popular filler materials are flour, fine sand, or other granular material. Don't use a liquid. You might think that this will make them more realistic and pliable but if your boobs get squeezed, you trip and bump them, or get squashed in the daily commute they may just pop on you. Having a suddenly flat boob is embarrassing but not as embarrassing as a slow leak that makes it look as though you are lactating.

Obviously, we want the right weight, pliability, smoothness, and bounciness. Depending on the weight of the material you might not be able to get the cup size you want without being too heavy or too light. Uncooked rice is just about the right consistency. Not only is the weight about right but when it is packed in it still has a certain squidge. For a holder you can use a plastic bag or balloon but both of these can make you sweat when they contact the skin. Although they do give some stickability onto your chest. An alternative which you'll have easy to hand is a pair of old stockings. If you use tights cut the panty bit off so you have two legs. Make sure the fabric matches to your skin tone. If your filler is lighter than your skin use a darker stocking so that they match up when the material gets tight and stretched.

Weigh out the right amount of material for one breast. Take a stocking and fill it with the right amount of rice or pop your already filled bag or balloon inside. Put your hand around the stocking and then trace down to the toe to pack the rice (or whatever) in good and firm. When you are happy with the feel, twist the stocking several times and then fold the whole lot inside itself. Now, smooth down, twist again and fold. Repeat this process until you have just enough material left to tie a knot. Repeat and you have your breast forms. Slip them into your bra and adjust. Put on a blouse or shirt and check the profile and movement.

If you are more adventurous the knot can be your nipple. Think about how big you want the nipple to be. knot and tie the remaining stocking a couple of times. If you need more bulk or want a more erect feel wrap something hard like a chickpea into some cotton wool and insert it into the stocking after the last twist and tie. Now twist again (just the nipple bit) and then tie the knot fitting any excess material over the nipple bump to make an areola. Now pop them in your bra and you're done.

What weight should you use? Well it depends on your cup size. Using the true sizes in the previous section and the weight of real women's breasts we get 32A = 0.5 pound per breast, 34B=0.7, 36C = 1.2, 38D = 1.7, and topping out at about 2 pounds per breast. That means that the average woman, 36C, carries about 2.4 pounds of weight on her chest. Use the same weight for a sister size – so 34B, 32C, 30D, and 36A all have the same weight of 0.7 pounds per breast. If you are not a true size the weight varies around the true size weight, for example: 34A = 0.6, 34B = 0.7 (the true size), 34C=0.9, 34D=1.5.

Think of the cone we used earlier. If you reduce the height of the cone the weight reduces. If the height increases the weight goes up. But this is not a linear scale. Breast weight increases faster as you go up from a true size than it decreases if your go down. The sister size stays the same because they all have the same volume. Get the idea? Measure some rice for the nearest true size to your desired breast and add or remove until you get something that has a reasonable fit with your bra cup. In fact, you can use the bra cup as a measuring spoon and then add or remove rice as needed.

Padding

The previous section assumes that you are flat chested and so have nothing to work with. If you have some breast development or man-boobs you can use fillets or other padding to round out your existing shape. The advantage of this approach is that with the right bra type you'll be able to show a natural cleavage and so wear a wider range of outfits.

The key to padding is to remember that boobs have to hang naturally with gravity so don't over stuff them to make them too pointy, perky, hard or round. The nipples of real breasts point horizontal or slightly down not up to the ceiling. We want to cushion and support the boobs. To see how this works, cup your breast material, with the hollow of the palm under the breast and the heel and thumb pad at the side against the rib. Now push inwards and lift the breasts. Notice how they look fuller. This is what we achieve with padding.

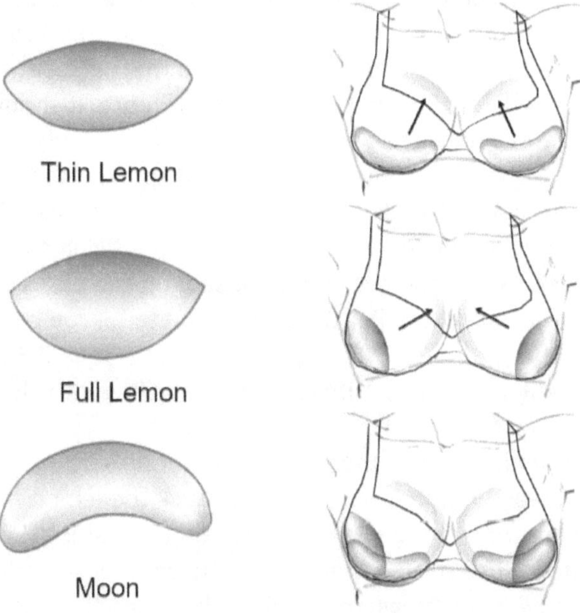

Figure 6 padding to enhance your bust

To pad effectively we use two types of padding a lemon and a moon shape (See Figure 6). Again, you can buy ready-made silicone ones or bra fillers but can also make your own. Often these are called fillets because they look and feel like a piece of uncooked chicken breast. The lemon fits in the side to give you fullness there. The moon is like a padded crescent shape and fits under the curve of your breast like the hollow of your hand to give lift and fullness there. The idea is that you take what breast material you have and push it up using the moon and then push it inwards from the side with the lemon. Once inside the bra these two things create a little cushion for your own breast tissue to sit on like a ledge which will give you extra plumpness and more importantly leave real flesh at the inner edge of the cups. Perfect!

DIY padding: lemons, moons and other sorts of pads can be bought quite easily at the local bra shop and also ordered on-line. Cheap ones cost only a few dollars. You can also buy inexpensive foam padding which fit inside the bra cups to bulk you up. Some people like to sew the padding into their everyday bras so that they don't have to fiddle with them when they are getting dressed.

Making your own padding is a cinch if you can hold a needle and thread. It can even be a girly pastime while you are enjoying some time en-femme. To make the moon use the circular edge of your bra cup and trace it onto a piece of card. The idea is you want a thin crescent shape. For the lemon use the side of the cup to taper that off more. It should look like an elongated lemon, hence the name.

For each shape cut out two identical shaped pieces of material and sew them together leaving one side open to make a pocket. Choose a plain washable fabric so they last a long time. Add the filling so that the pad is gently rounded like a little cushion. Now sew up the pocket. Make two of each, one for each bra cup. For the padding material you can use foam cut to size, or batting folded to the right thickness – tack it together in the shape you want with a few stitches before stuffing into the pocket. That way it will be easier to handle.

Put on your bra and then insert the moon into the cup tucking it under what breast material you have then tuck the lemon into the side to get a nice shape. Adjust the sit of your own breast material in the top of the cup and then the bra strap as necessary. The amount of padding you need depends on how much breast material you have and the size of the cup you want. Test that out by sticking something like a sock in the cup as a pad first to get the sit you want and then use that thickness of padding to make your lemon and moon.

Because the padding is hidden inside the cups and not usually visible this means that you can be more flexible about what you wear. For example, lower cut dresses or V-necks where a little of the cleavage is visible. You can also indulge yourself with nice lacy bras to show off your décolletage (shoulders and or lower neckline) to best advantage.

The main problem with padding is that the pads can be quite lightweight. Either you live with it or make a little insert with heavier material and wrap it in the stuffing to get a soft weight. You can use the scale above for the weight but remember to deduct off the weight of your own boob material. To do this weigh your own boob using the displacement method and then subtract the result from your desired breast weight.

If all this seems like too much effort an easier approach is to make a padded bra. For this you'll need some foam of the same thickness that you want to pad – that is the difference between your own bust measurement and the one you want to be. Insert the foam into the bra cup (while you're not wearing it) and then press it smooth. Trace the outline of the cup on the foam with a marker pen then extract the foam and cut out the shape. You can also buy pads like this for relatively low cost. Use these as inserts or sew the whole pad into the cup so the bra is always properly padded.

Au-natural (or the art of taping)

The final method of constructing a breast shape doesn't use padding or forms at all. The secret to this kind of structure is strapping or tape. Because there is no bra you can wear backless dresses or one-piece swimsuits, loose baggy shirts or blouses, rompers, or nighties and still feel natural.

Everyone evolves their own little tricks on how to tape because we all have different shapes. But what you need is a good roll of adhesive tape that will stick to the skin. Some common choices are medical tape, athletic tape, or cloth tape specifically designed for breast taping. Duct taping will work but is a devil to remove and irritates sensitive skin. Check that you are not allergic to Elastoplast or the kind of adhesive on the tape you are using. Also, there is an assumption that you are clean shaven on the chest and back area. Otherwise its going to get painful and messy when it comes to pulling off the tape.

The tapes do the job of lifting the breast up and pulling it in towards the middle of your chest. We'll look at two methods one with four pieces of tape and one with six. Once you get the idea it's not difficult.

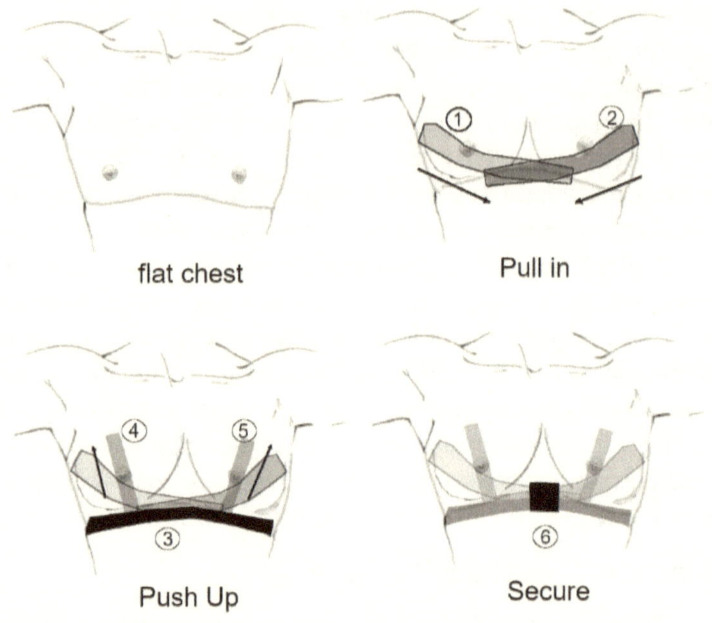

Figure 7 Taping to make a bigger bust

In the four-piece method you want two smaller strips about the diameter of your cup size plus a bit extra. These will act like fillets. Then a longer piece about half your band size (to fit only your front). And a smaller bit to hold it all together. Take the first 'fillet' strip and attach it level to your breast under the arm pit. Pull it tight across the side of your boob and pull inwards and fix the tape under the boob on the opposite side towards the centre of your chest. Do the same with the second tape on the other side. Now take the longer chest piece and attach it like the band of your bra under the front of your boobs and over the end of the side tapes to stop them pulling away. Pull the band in from both sides to give a snug fit and use the fourth piece of tape to secure any excess between your boobs. Wrap it around and then stick down where the cleavage would be making a little cross. Make it as short as possible so you have the option to show a bit of cleavage if you want to.

The six-piece method is similar except you need two extra pieces of tape to help lift the breast. Secure the fillet tapes as in the previous method. Now take one of the extra bits and attach it under the centre of your boob on the ribcage and run it up and over, pull to get a lift and snug fit then tape it to the upper chest. Repeat for the other boob. Now attach the band tape making sure it lays over both the fillet and bottom end of the chest tape. Then secure the excess as you pull in the boobs as for the four-piece methods. Depending on how secure you feel you might want to add more tapes either sideways or vertically. For example, using three vertical strips at different points along the chest can make an acceptable cup to give the lower portion of the breast more support.

Another popular variation for a no-bra look in t-shirts (anything with a back) is to simply take a roll of tape and attach under the armpit at nipple level then wrap it around the torso making sure you pull your boobs in on the first pass to get a tight fit. This is pretty much a modern-day version of chest binding popular with Roman women. The idea was to make their boobs smaller, perkier, and rounder on the cleavage. You can also go around the back with the previous methods if you aren't wearing anything backless. There are many variations on this idea.

The fake cleavage

The degree to which you squeeze your puppies up and inwards using your bra straps or tape will make a natural cleavage. The width of your chest will determine how voluptuous this little valley appears. If you still have a sizable gap between one side and the other (say more than an inch) then you can use this little trick to appear more fulsome.

The fake cleavage is an optical illusion. It uses the principle of depth perception that artists employ to get a three-dimensional image on a flat canvas. In this case it is your flatter chest we are working on. If we think about how light bounces off an object then there are three types of shade (or value) full light, mid tone, and shadow. As things move from being in full light to shadow the value of the colour of the object gets darker. So, if we think of your chest and cleavage the top of your boob is in full light and then darkens as it goes into the crease. If your boobs are closer together you'll get a darker shadow than if they are far apart. And, if they are almost touching, you'll get a narrow little line (called the horizon – even though it is vertical) where everything is black because no light can get in to be reflected.

What we want to do is recreate this effect on your chest. The way we do this is by using makeup. In particular, a palette of colours you use on your face to get contours and definition for your cheeks. Starting with your natural skin tone (of your chest area) choose a darker one and then a mid-tone in between. Tape up or pad your boobs and get the best cleavage you can. Now brush in the colour in a semi-circular shape between each breast in the cleavage area and work the material to make a nice contour. Work on this to blend it in to the contour of your existing bust so that there is a smooth transition. Et volia! Now you have a neat looking deeper cleavage.

All this can take a little practice. Make a copy of the first picture in Figure 7 and fill in the boobs by shading with a pencil. This will give you an idea of the shape and degree of shading required to get a realistic looking pair of well-developed breasts. Figure 6 shows you what a little shading looks like on the cleavage area. If you are artistic job done. Then go to colour so that you can work more on the tone and blending. Subtle is often more effective. And don't forget the boob shadow under your breast material that has that crescent moon shape. Extending here can make you look fuller and heavier.

The trick is not to go too dark on the colours. If you have a one-inch gap, a half inch on each side is enough to leave a hint of a gap between. If you a wider than an inch don't infill too much. Take about an inch and half from each boob inwards. The wider your final cleavage the less dark the crease should be in the middle. Maybe even just a hint of shadow. If you are wider than two inches taping isn't really working for you. Look for another method to create your boobs.

At a distance it will look very effective, but the illusion disappears the closer you get to someone. Done well you can be standing in conversation with another person and they won't be able to tell that its fake. If you want to be more intimate or undress obviously your secret will be revealed. But if your objective is social dressing or a night out for fun it can be a good option. A fake cleavage looks better in a nightclub where the lighting is already subdued. Experts, like drag queens, can get away with it on stage in bright lights.

Top Tip: use makeup fixer after you get the right look. If you are partying and perspiring, you don't want to be smudging down there. This is worse than your mascara running when you cry. Plus, you don't want to mess up a pretty or light-coloured bra with rub off. Makeup can be a pain to get off clothing. And nothing worse than under things looking a bit grubby.

Bra types

Our next topic is Bra types. There are upwards of twenty different shapes and style of bra some functional, some pretty and fashionable, and some for naughty fun. Generally, the support you get reduces the more fashionable or fun the bra. Some sexy lingerie is more about presenting your boobs rather than supporting and looking after them. So apart from a standard bra which you should always have in your closet here are four types that will give you a different look and allow you to experiment with all sorts of clothing.

Type 1: functional –Under wire, fuller figure, Sports, racer back, multiway

The functional bras are all designed to help support the bust. The under-wire bra has a length of wire or resin sewn into the bottom half of the cup to give more support for the breast cup. If your cup size is greater than a B then you should consider this sort of arrangement. To have a fuller figure your cup size must be a D or greater. The fuller figure bra has bigger and more robust cups to hold the extra weight. Problem is they look a bit retro or matronly so what you get in support you lose in prettiness. There are some lacy ones out there if you look in plus sized stores.

The sports bras are more substantial with bigger bands and shoulder straps designed to stop things moving too much while you exercise. A sports bra has the traditional shoulders whereas in a racer-back the straps join in the centre of the back. If you don't like the straps of your bra showing in sleeveless tops or dresses pin or tie them together to form an improvised fashion racer-back and avoid the problem. In a multiway there are several smaller straps to help support breast weight and movement but they are also adjustable so you can wear them as a regular over the shoulder style or crossed over the back or both.

Type 2: playful - pushup , plunge, balconette, cage

The next set still offer some support but are more playful or flirty. A push up is a fashion bra that has angled and padded cups to push the breasts inwards and upwards to create a cleavage. It may incorporate under wiring as well to support bigger boobs. A demi-cup (or half to three quarter cup) is often used which exposes more of the breast tissue. Consequently, great for low tops or off-the-shoulder style clothes.

A plunge bra has a deeper cut in the gore (or bridge section between the cups). The deeper cleavage means you can wear plunge necklines and V-shaped tops. The balconette or balcony bra has a demi-cup but is flatter with the cup more horizontal. This creates a cleavage and still covers the nipple while showing more of the upper breast. Normally the straps are more to the side. The bra is higher there and it looks like the boobs are on a shelf. Use this type for low cut squared tops or peasant style blouses.

The cage bra on the other hand includes a cup and some extra strapping over the breasts. The cups can be missing while still giving some sort of support if you want a more racy bondage feel (and of course have some breast material).

Type 3: cute- trainer, bralette, halter, T-shirt

The trainer bra is not really a bra in that it doesn't support anything it just looks like a bra. Young girls wear trainers to get used to the feel of a bra and to cover sensitive budding and nipple areas. If you are in a female led relationship or undergoing feminization your partner or mistress may put you into a trainer as a first step or as a teasing exercise to emphasise your small man boobs. Some may have slogans or other girly motifs – like princess, or rainbows, unicorns or other cute animals.

The bralette is another bra like item that doesn't provide support and is more useful for smaller cup-sizes (A and small B's). The bralette is more like a top or prettier sports bra. Sometimes a bralette will have a little bit of padding to cover the nipple area for modesty. Use them like a crop-top or if you want to show something under looser clothing that is not a full bra.

A halter bra is more like a sleeveless top with some shaping over the breasts. The straps are connected behind the neck rather than over the shoulder. Thus, the bra can be worn with halter style dresses or tops.

The T-shirt bra has very smooth cups with most of the seams removed or pushed to the side (or wings) of the bra band. They can also incorporate some padding. This allows them to be worn under very tight-fitting clothing (like T-shirts) without any unsightly bumps and lines. Use these bras if you want to look as though you aren't wearing a bra.

Type 4: revealing – strapless, tube, bridal, stick-on,

The next set of bras are all designed so that you can wear off-the-shoulder outfits that show most of your torso from the neck to the bust. The strapless bra achieves this by not having any strap attachments and stiffer cups. The band is often thicker and more substantial because it is doing all the support. Women often go down a band size and increase the cup so that the band is tighter and holds the breasts which are pushed up for a voluptuous look suitable for evening gowns.

A tube bra is a strapless strip of stretchy fabric with a thick band on the top and bottom for better hold. Normally they come with removable pads but that is all the support you get. The Bandeau variation simply wraps around your boobs with no support other than the tightness of material.

A bridal bra is an extension of the strapless idea with the band area extended down the ribcage to form a bustier. This look is popular with brides-to-be because it allows low cut and off the shoulder dresses to be worn but can also be pretty with lots of lace finish on the extended band. Sometimes the band at the back is also lowered or shaped to allow for backless dresses.

The stick-on bra is like a strapless bar but is usually consists of just the cups and gore. They are made of some sort of silicone and may have padding. The insides of the cups are coated with adhesive that sticks onto the breasts. They can give you the advantages of a push up while also appearing as though you are braless and come in a variety of designs. Some crossdressers with a little breast material use the stick-on as an alternative to taping for that au-natural look.

Shopping list

Okay here's the shopping list for this chapter. You don't need all the things on this list so choose what is in your budget or the look you want.

Athletic, body or boob Tape (quite cheap for 5m or multiple tapes)
Padding (foam lemons and moons are cheap, silicone a bit more expensive, 10 pounds/dollars)
Breast forms (not cheap at 100-200 dollars/pounds).
Pocket bras (to hold your breast forms 20 dollars/pounds upwards)
Harness bras with boob attachments (20 dollars/pounds upwards)
Sensible bras –10 or under, 20/30 dollar/pounds
Lingerie, designer, and fashion bras and push ups 40-50 dollar/pounds upwards
Face makeup palette and brush set and remover if you don't already have them.
A bag or two of rice and a pair of stockings can be affordable in your weekly shop.

When ordering breast forms, you'll need to know the look and type you want (e.g. silicon, with nipple detail etc), plus the width, length, and height that fit your chest. Often the weight of the form is given as well. You might notice they are a little light compared to our measurements this is because they assume that you have some fatty breast material already. Take this into account or ask when ordering.

An alternative coverall is a silicone crop top with inbuilt breasts. This is like a little flesh coloured sleeveless vest for the upper body. It solves the whole chest area problem but retails in the region of 500-700 pounds/dollars. You don't even have to shave your chest though you'll get a better fit if you do.

And finally ...

Again, much to think about here in terms of options and what you are willing to spend. As a general rule, though, the less natural options like breast forms will restrict to some extent whether you can be intimate. If you are just socialising or dressing for an everyday look then fine.

The more you use your natural gifts you'll have to look after the skin more (see the chapter on pampering). The best way to remove taping is to immerse in warm water till the adhesive lifts and you can just peel it off. After a night out or a period of dressing it is a good idea to have some personal time for a bath. Likewise, if you have made a work of art out of your cleavage, you'll need to remove that with makeup removal products. Moisturise to keep everything healthy.

Last but not least. If you are looking for intimacy and sensual play, then forget all the boob stuff and just buy some pretty small cup (A or B) bras and lingerie (see later). If you shave your chest and have some material there, even if it is just fatty, you can use makeup to give some nipple detail or a little hint at boobs and feel girly while indulging your other needs.

Chapter 6 Butts and other Bits

The lower part of your torso is the next area of consideration. We are going to look at both the front and back. In the latter we want a nice round or pert female bottom that looks good in all sorts of outfits and in the former that nice little Y shape that you see in swimwear and lingerie photoshoots.

The bottom area can set off your figure and attract attention when you bend, twist, stretch or reach over for things. That important little curve between the small of your back and the bottom also dictates how a dress or skirt will fall around your legs or off your hips. The shape of your bottom will also contribute to or lessen the chance of visible panty lines if you wear business suits, pant suits, or other tight fighting things.

In the front area we are talking about how to hide your male bits. There probably isn't a crossdresser alive that hasn't stood naked in front of a full-length mirror and tucked the Johnson between their legs and posed like a girl. Well, if you want to stay that way for an extended period without aches or pains or be able to move and pose there is an art to it. We'll look at all that in the following sections along with some health advice.

Butt types

Not all butts are the same. You knew that, right? The shape of your posterior is a combination of your hip structure, how wide you are, and the fullness of your bottom cheeks. The cheek or glutinous maximus is an area of fatty tissue that covers the vital nerves and muscles running from your spine down the legs so that they don't get damaged when we sit or bump ourselves.

If your bot is round, curvy or pert it can be very sexy. A designer bottom makes a person want to touch it, feel its roundness, smoothness, hold it or indeed spank it. And, it will also play a part in how good you look in lingerie. All things considered, worth a bit of attention. The types of outfits you wear and of course that most intimate of female garments panties depend on the shape of your butt whether it is to just to feel sexy and comfortable, show off your cheeks, or avoid visible panty lines.

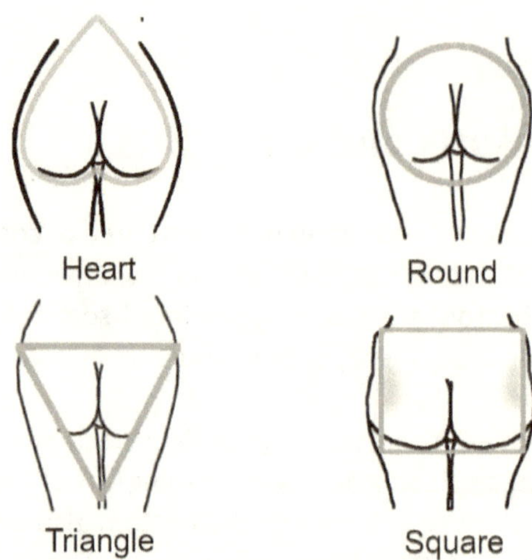

Figure 8 Bottom shapes

Just like our body, butts can be divided into types. There are four major categories; heart, round, square, and triangle (see Figure 8). Let's look at each of these.

Heart: this is best described as an upside-down heart shape with the point at the centre of your back just above the pelvis (where there are often two dimples) and the round bits tracing the outline of your hips and cheeks. The weight of the bottom is lower down in the cheeks which are wider but tapers upwards. Typically, it fits with a pear-shape figure where the hips are wider. Hence the idea that pear-shape bottoms are big.

Round: the round bottom fits inside a circle centred on the point where the bottom cheeks separate. It is widest at the hips. The bottom cheeks are contained inside the lower half of the circle and the upper part marks the start of the waist. The fat in the cheeks is more rounded and evenly distributed either side of the vertical centre line of the circle and projects out more which gives this style the alternative name of bubble-butt.

Triangle: in this bottom shape the widest part is at the top of the hips just before the waist and tapers down towards the centre of the butt crack but extends beyond it to form an upside triangle. The bottom cheeks are defined by the tapering and so are narrower than the hips. The fat material is mostly at the top of the bottom with the cheeks smaller and flatter at the sides. This is the bottom most associated with the broad shoulders of a strawberry shape and is a typical man bot but is also surprisingly common amongst female models. Maybe because it can easily appear cute and pert.

Square: here the hips do not taper as much as the above types so that the hip and bottom stay in line giving a straight vertical between the hip and the top of the legs. The cheeks lie inside the bottom edge of a square defined by the top of the hips and the top of the thigh. The weight here is evenly distributed but may not look as curvy as the other butt types. You may also see a depression or dimple between the hip and the face of the bottom cheek. This type is often associated with the rectangle shape but the dimples can also make you look skinny.

Because men have small less rounded pelvic bones the chances are that your butt type is either triangle or square. If you are adding hip padding to create a curvier silhouette, then you'll have to think about matching that with some adjustments to your butt. Adding some padding to the lower portion of the cheek can easily create more roundness and lift suitable for either type 1 or type 2. Adding some side cheek padding can fill out the square shape and also make you rounder as in type 2 or work with any waist reduction to create a more type 1 heart shape.

All this can be achieved using control panties (see foundation wear). Then adding your choice of fashion pantie over the top. Usually the best pantie will be a fuller pant to cover your foundation garment but they can still be pretty and silky or sheer fabric. If you want to be more intimate and feel the softness of the pantie material or pretty-it-up with lacy and daring cuts then the good news is that with some imagination you can find pretty panties to suit each of these butts and avoid the padding.

The best panties for your type

Unlike male pants that are confined to two or three basic cuts there are upwards of nine different styles of pantie.

For everyday use there are the classic pantie (or brief), the high cut brief, or control pants. These are often referred to by a woman has her big pants and not seen as necessarily sexy although they can be pretty in a girl-next-door kind of way. Think Bridget Jones's diary.

The next set of three are hipsters, bikini, and boy shorts which are a little sexier but can still be used for every day. The higher cuts and waist bands allow some pretty lace detail and patterning whereas the first three are usual plain cotton or silk.

The last three cuts are Tanga, Thong, and G-string. These are skimpy panties and often reveal a lot of the bottom cheeks and are matched up with pretty bras and things in lingerie. They can give the no pants feel and are usually of very flimsy material that barely covers the front.

Although all these pantie cuts are very feminine the latter are often considered more girly. You might think they are impossible for anyone with bits other than female, but you'd be wrong. More on that later. Let's look at each type of bottom and choose the best pantie style.

The heart shape lends itself to thongs and G-strings which emphasise those lovely cheeks by highlighting the top half to counterbalance the wide bottom areas. Use lacy frills, ruffles and ruches to pull the eye upwards and give extra perkiness. Bikinis also work but be cautious of anything with solid colour that will make you look wider. For the fuller style pants choose a thinner material, pastels if you want colour and higher cut legs. Small leg opening will bunch up the material and it will end up in the butt crease. Tighter elasticated material can also help firm up your bottom and pull in the heart shape a little if you think it is too wide.

The round shape has more width across the centre and has more volume so fuller pants are tricky to get the coverage and bikini styles will tend to bite into the cheek and form panty lines because of the fullness. Most of the roundness comes out at the middle of the cheek. The trick is to go with a high cut pantie so that the material gathers towards the top of the hip and sides to leave a nice round line over the side of the cheek. What you want to avoid is excess fabric. Choose things that are not as elasticated (as they will tend to dig into your more rounded parts) but still give nice coverage.

The Triangle shape creates a different challenge. Here we have less roundness and width at the bottom. Use a smaller leg cut to bring material down over your bottom cheeks. Choose ones that bring the leg in under the butt cheeks close to the crease. You can fool the eye into thinking there is more fullness by choosing panties with lacy and frill detail on the leg openings or across the lower bottom. A boy short or standard pantie is a good choice with solid colour and/or lace patterns to again give the impression of more butt volume. With a fuller pant you have the option of some side padding to round out the flatness. A rhumba or layered style will also make you rounder and more heart shaped.

The square is the final shape and perhaps the trickiest since it can appear that your bottom is non-existent. The trick here is to simulate roundness. Go for a higher waist band to show where your bottom starts. Use the higher leg cuts to emphasise curves on the sides. And, whereas you want solid colours on the triangle to push the butt out here you want to avoid those to curve the butt in. Choose things with lacy swirls or patterns. Showing a little bit more of the lower cheek as in boy shorts also tends to suggest a heart shape.

So, the factors to consider are the size of leg opening, the cut on the hip (low or high), whether you want to display the bottom cheeks or not, plus the level of pretty detail with lace, ruffles, and layers.

Butt pads and lifting

We looked at foundation wear and padding in the previous chapter. Still it is worth a few more words on the particulars of butt augmentation.

If what your need is a lift of your existing butt cheeks. For example, with a heart shape or a saggy square shape you can bring the flexible glutinous maximus up into a firmer configuration with control pants that leave the area open but have extended and strong elastic under the curve of the cheek. This configuration puts the fleshy material into a more rounded position. On the other hand, if the problem is flat side cheeks as in square or triangle shape a fillet is used to pad out the depression and give you fullness and roundness there. If your bottom is just flat overall, you can give it some curve at the bottom with some moon shaped pads under the cheeks to give a shape more like the heart and round types. See Figure 9 for some examples. If you are going to pad then it makes sense to create a more female shaped bottom like a type 1 or type 2.

Because you will be sitting on the pads quite a lot it is better if the padding is woven or sewn into the pantie. This means that you can wear your control panties and then pull on bigger pants over the top and complement it with other padding solutions for the hips and thighs. You can get lifting pants from women's shops and pads from specific crossdressing outlets.

If you find you like your new butt shape you can always consider making it permanent with a cosmetic procedure. A butt lift will raise the cheeks. An implant will put medical grade pads inside your body. And liposuction can move fat from your other places to your butt. One reason to consider this is that obviously you can do away with your pads and just choose the panties you like. Another is that with padding you will be less sensitive to touch. So, if someone does take a fancy to you and decides to fondle or pinch your tush you won't feel it. That means that you won't necessarily be able to appreciate it or to reprimand the person doing the touching.

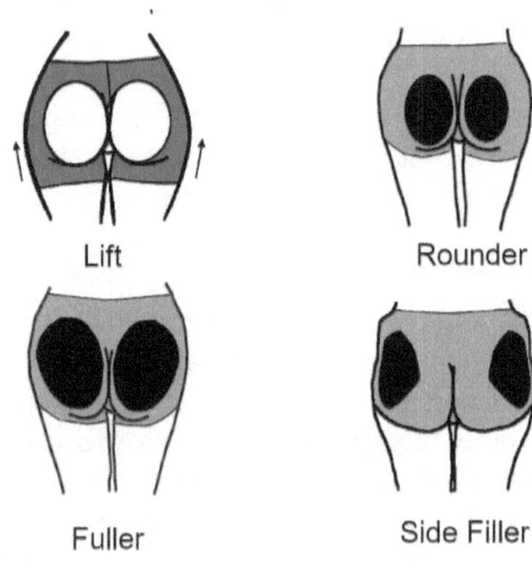

Figure 9 Enhancing the bottom with padding

One final word on butt padding. Too much pressure on your cheeks can compress the sciatic nerves that run from your spine down into your legs. If you damage this area you will end up with a tingling sensation or ache in your lower legs. Men that carry their wallets in their back pockets often suffer from this and it can be exhausting. It shouldn't be a problem if your pads fit properly and don't shift about. Make sure your shapewear is tight enough to hold them in place but not so tight that it causes irritation or digs into the skin. You shouldn't stay dressed for too long without relief if you have significant butt padding. This could be a problem if, say, you have a desk job and sit a lot. In that case just select nice panties using the guide above.

Pocketing

Now let's turn to the front. Before we can get into tucking proper there a few things you should know about your anatomy that may surprise you.

First off, your body still has the remnants of when you were growing in the womb before your turned into a boy. Both males and females have a set of tubing called the inguinal canals. In the female they connect to the womb (uterus) and run down to the pubic area near the major labia (or lips). In the male they run from the same area near the kidneys and into the pubic area.

Before we develop ovaries or testicles, we all have the same kind of gland called a gonad which either stays where it is (female and becomes an ovary) or drops down the inguinal canal (male and becomes a testicle). The trick to hiding your testicles is to place your balls back in these tubes which are still inside your body.

The inguinal canals lie either side of your penis and if you take a testicle and push it gently back and up towards your body there is a little pocket. Depending on your size the testicle should more or less pop inside again without too much difficulty. Keep your hand in place next to your crotch and allow the testicle to find a happy natural position. It should feel comfortable. If it aches or bulges under your skin, you have pushed a little too far. There is a little constriction along the canal which will stop you losing the testicle altogether. You'll find that it you let go it will pop back out again. The art in pocketing is to place your balls in the pockets and then find a way to stop them dropping out.

The cremaster muscle

When we are born the testicles are inside the body. Only later do they drop down into the scrotum (or ball sac). They come out of the body so that they can stay at the right temperature to encourage testosterone and sperm production. The testicles start in the abdomen and move down the inguinal canal to a place just inside the body called the inguinal pouch ready to drop out of the body into the ball sac. All this happens when we are babies.

Once in the scrotum the testicle rests in another pouch like structure called the cremaster muscle. This muscle pulls the testicle closer to the body when we exercise, for protection, to regulate temperature or get ready for orgasm. If the cremaster reflex is strong it can pull the testicle all the way back into the inguinal pouch. Supposedly martial artists can learn to do this at will in a technique called iron groin. When they get kicked between the legs it doesn't hurt. Bet you never thought you'd be learning kung fu as part of your dressing.

The cremaster muscle holds your testicles in place and can lift them closer to the body. Normally this is an involuntary reaction but with persistence it can be controlled. You can get this reaction easily by softly stroking your inner thigh from just above the knee to just below the crotch.

A woman well versed in the erotic arts knows how to stroke you in this way. They know that as the balls come up you will get more turned-on and can tease or edge you. A female dominant may do that but also add an element of humiliation by pointing out that you are shrinking or turning into a girl. Fear and laughter also work. As does a cold shower!

If you want to learn to control this reflex the following exercises will strengthen the cremaster muscles. First is to gently pull the balls and scrotum down and away from your body. Not too far, just to get a tension in the muscle. Next squeeze your pubococcygeus (PC) muscle. This muscle connects your pubic bone to the bottom of the spine. You squeeze this to stop yourself urinating when you are caught short and you might find that your anus contracts as well. This exercise also contracts the cremaster muscle. If you want a more girly exercise Kegel (pelvic floor) exercises also work as does contracting your abdominal muscles. You might only notice a little movement to begin with but it should develop with time. Do a few repetitions every day. For example, when you wake up in the morning, before you go to sleep, or are in the bath.

In tucking we want your balls in the pouch not shoved up too far into the inguinal canal. Once in this position you will have to be a little gentle on movement but hey, that's a good thing, it will make you more lady-like. As a rule, if you start to feel a dull ache you have been in the position too long. That applies to all these tucking techniques. If you find it is too uncomfortable, your testicles are too big for the pouch, or you just don't fancy the idea there are other ways to tuck that don't need this step.

Contrary to common urban myths ejaculating does not change your testicle size. The contribution of the testicle is only about 3% of the total volume of any fluid emitted. Tucking will not get easier if you do this beforehand. In fact, probably it will be worse because as soon as you have emptied chemical signals put your testicles into sperm production mode making them more sensitive.

Taking hormones like estrogen and steroids in the long run produces smaller, less active, pre-pubescent balls which then become easier to pocket. So, if you are on HRT or transitioning or do a lot of weight training and bulk up using steroids eventually you should be able to pocket and hide the testicles completely.

The average size of your plums are 1.8-2 inches in length with anything below 1.4 being considered small and above 2 as larger. It is not unusual for one testicle to be a little larger than the other (usually the right one) which may affect how you arrange things when you tuck. But if there is a big difference and they are sensitive go see a doctor.

If you have frequent erections without ejaculating your testicles will get a little bigger. This is a temporary condition called epididymal hypertension (or blue balls) caused by expansion of blood vessels in preparation for erection. When the blood is not released by orgasm it can cause pain, discomfort, heaviness, or aching. This occurs if you are easily aroused or if you play edging games. So be careful with pocketing and tucking if this is what you want to do while dressed.

Finally, if the cremaster muscle gets too strong it can retract the testicle permanently a condition called ascending testicle. This might sound like a good idea from your femme perspective but if it happens you should seek medical help as it can become chronic and debilitating. Occasionally the cremaster can cramp causing a painful spasm and not release. If this happens take a warm bath to help it relax. If it doesn't release go to the doctor. As we get older though the muscle weakens so it may drop in and out periodically.

The art of Tucking

Now we get to tucking proper. Tucking is another of those love it or hate things. If your objective is arousal when you dress, why would you want to tuck and make access difficult? If you tuck and go out, you'll have to think about how to use toilets and so forth as well as having extra tape and things in your bag so you can redo the tuck. With body contoured outfits or tight pencil skirts you'll want to avoid a little tell-tale lump at an inconvenient location. If your look is petticoats and fuller skirts or dresses tucking won't matter that much. Then again, if you identity strongly as female, having something dangling will be a constant distraction and reminder of maleness.

The basics: Tucking has four basic steps. How far you go depends on how well endowed you are and what you want to do when dressed. Just so you know the average size of a flaccid penis is 3.5 inches and when erect 5.1 inches. Statistically flaccid size is not a good predictor of erect size. Anything over six inches is considered big and lower than 5 inches is considered small. A micro-penis is anything less than 3 inches. In 'forced' feminization literature these small sizes are referred to as dicklets or sissy clits. Most people should be able to tuck the average size but if you are bigger you might need more fastening and if smaller there are some particularly girly options.

The four steps are pocketing, wrapping, folding, and fastening. Pocketing as above refers to hiding your testicles in your body this makes them less obvious and can avoid inadvertently squeezing them and causing pain when you move around while they are tucked. Wrapping refers to bandaging the penis in some manner so that it can be held in place and not damaged by any methods of fastening. Folding refers to hiding the penis or testicles or both between the legs. And, last is fastening which uses tape or other methods to stop your tuck from coming undone or moving around and causing problems while you are dressed.

Wrapping the penis involves encasing the shaft in some material so that it can be held and pulled into a final resting place of the tuck. There are two main ways to do this. First is to use some soft cloth or lint and tape it around the penis so that it won't easily slip off. That is easier said than done. Some people just make a little bag or pouch for the penis and tie it in place around the testicles which is possible if you do not pocket. The trick is to tape firmly enough to get a hold of the penis but not so tight that you lose circulation.

Some practitioners simply use athletic or medical tape directly on the skin to wrap. This avoids slippage but can irritate and pull the flesh if you stay tucked for a long time. Another alternative if you are on the smaller side is to use the empty scrotum (assuming you have pocketed). Wrap either sides of the empty bag around the penis and then tape around. If you are inventive you can arrange it so the head of the penis is close to an opening in the wrap to make a faux clitoris. This also makes it easier to urinate while tucked.

Whatever wrapping technique is used you want the binding firm but not so tight that it cuts off the circulation. If you are going to be tucked for a while it is good practice to check regularly to ensure everything is healthy. And to loosen things up periodically to allow proper circulation. If anything looks purple or bluish time for a rest. Also give yourself plenty of time when you are not tucked to maintain everything in good condition and avoid complications. Always spend more time untucked than tucked.

Armed with these two techniques of pocketing and wrapping we can tuck in a variety of ways by folding and fastening. Since we will be using tape and such like it is easier to tuck in more advanced positions if your genitals and peri-anal area are clean shaven and smooth so that things will stick and are easier to remove. Remember we are using medical or athletic tape which is designed to stick to skin. When you do want to remove the fastening do it gently. Preferably take a warm bath and let it all soak to loosen up the adhesive so it peels off more easily. Moisturise the skin and/or apply some talc to keep things healthy afterwards as part of your pamper routine.

Basic folding: in this technique we don't do anything sophisticated. All you need is a pair of control panties. Put the panties on and pull them up to mid-thigh. Fold your genitals between your legs and arrange them comfortably and then pull up the panties fully. It is often easier to align the testicles one after the other and then penis alongside. This avoids too much pressure when you cross your legs girl fashion. Because the panties are elasticated, they will hold the tuck in place and with a control panel on the front will help flatten your pubic area into the female Y-shape. You can get a smoother profile if you pocket because this will leave more space for the penis to fold back between your legs. The problem though is that things might not feel all that secure and control panties aren't very pretty.

Using a Gaff: as an alternative buy some plain skimpy panties (e.g. bikini or tanga) that are quite well elasticated but get them one or two sizes too small. This will ensure a tight fit on the leg and hip. Proceed with a basic folding and the tighter material and gusset will hold the tuck in place. This is a popular technique because it allows you to wear what you want. Buy plain nude ones and then you can put a prettier fuller pantie over the top. A variation is a specially made type of support called a gaff. The gaff retains the elastic part of a panty and just enough gusset material to hold the tuck in place. A gaff can be purchased from most crossdressing stores. Some are fuller (tanga) in style but all give you the hold required to keep things in place. Alternatively make your own by cutting a smaller pair of control panties down to size. Keep the elastic for the legs and the gusset and sew waist elastic on top to make small skimpy control panties.

Basic Taping: with both the above methods you might find that you don't quite have that little pussy bump profile you see in swimsuit and underwear pictures. The reason is that when the penis bends the base and the shaft form a U-shape which sticks out a little. The bigger you are the more knuckle of the U-shaped fold will show. Wrap the penis and attach some tape lengthwise so you can pull the penis further back so that profile is flatter and more girlie. There are numerous ways to do this.

One method uses two lengths of tape long enough to attach onto your bottom cheeks (see Figure 10). Fix one end to the wrap and then pull back through the legs to get a secure fit and then tape under the curve of the bottom and up onto the cheek. This should help keep the testicles pocketed. Repeat for the other cheek. Add a strip around the wrap to stop the wrapping pulling off. For a more secure fit add a third piece of tape to run up between your bottom cheeks and secure just above the crease. Wrap a piece of cloth or other soft material around the place where the tape runs over the anus. If you stick the tape to this spot it will rub and irritate and be difficult to get off without damaging the sensitive skin. Extend the tape forward over the pubic area to give more support. Make a little fan shape of smaller tapes running up onto the pubis. This will give the wrap more security and allow a more pleasing pussy shape.

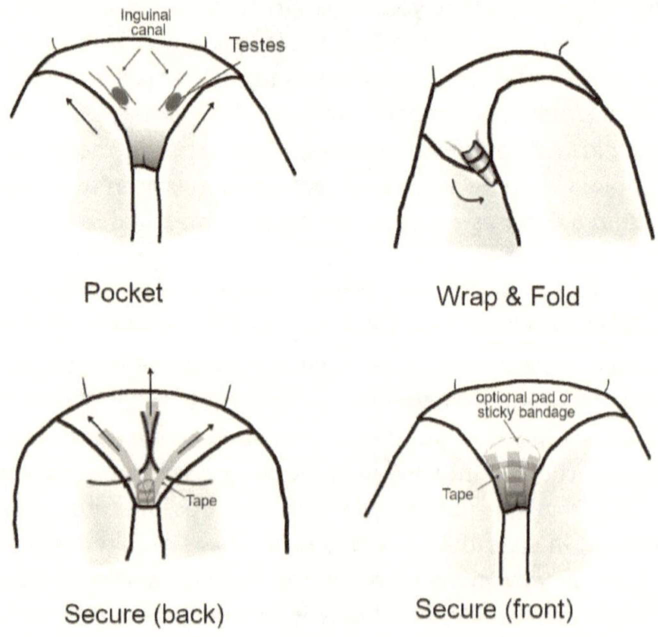

Figure 10 Tucking to create a smooth look

The advantage of all these taping methods is that you can wear a wider range of panties and nothing will show. Choose ones with thicker or more opaque material and wider gusset to hide the taping. The downside is of course that you're fixed. Going to the toilet requires you undo and then reapply the taping. And, of course, any sort of erotic play is out of the question.

Padding: sometimes you can get a more pleasing profile if you pad the pubic area. For this you'll need that eternally feminine product – a panty liner, sanitary towel, or incontinence pad. Choose a slim version with the rounded ends so it looks nice on the pubic area. These products are designed to have the absorbent parts against the vagina which is exactly where your fold ends up so they are a nice cushion. In this tuck you do the same as before but use the pad to hold the fold. The pad gives you greater surface area for any taping and you can position it over the folded penis to give the U-shape a smoother line. An advantage is that you are not taping or wrapping the penis so can avoid circulation issues.

Tape the front of the pad neatly to the pubic area so that the tape doesn't extend too far and restrict the type of panties you can wear. For best hold use a fan shape with tape running back under the legs. Also tape back up through the butt cheeks as in the previous methods. An added feature of this version is that it is more discreet when you go out and easier to redo. You will need to carry items to fix things when you go to the restroom. The extra pads won't draw attention if people do see inside your handbag because it has more feminine contents. They'll just think it is your time of the month which adds to your feminine mystique.

If your endowment is on the smaller side, you might not be able to fold or wrap at all. In this case pocket and then use a larger adhesive bandage to cover the whole arrangement. This avoids the padding altogether. Alternatively, if you have some fatty material on your pubis you can press the micro penis into towards the pubic bone. Usually there is enough soft tissue for the penis to sit in a little dimple and for the folds of skin to close over it to form a little slit. Cover the whole area with an adhesive bandage like a big plaster. Use a see-through version if you want the slit to be visible. If there is enough fatty material down there you can construct a small pussy slit and use less tape. Tape across the top of the join and let the head of the penis appear at the bottom half of the slit. Tape the bottom part underneath as well. This way you can make a faux clitoris while it is tucked. The sensitive head part of the penis can be stimulated, and it gives you a more female appearance.

Other methods: another approach is to use a female fashion accessory called a C-string. Basically, this is like a G-string but without a waist band. The front section covers the pubic area and a wired section runs between the legs and bottom cheeks to grip just where the crease of your bottom meets the back. The tension in the wire holds it in place. Use a pad or other wrap to cushion the genitals against the wire and then slip on the C-string to give you a nice front profile. A tip is to tape the padding to the C-string. That way it covers the tuck and is all easy to remove if you need to use the restroom. The C-string can then hide all traces and you can wear other panties over the top.

More expensive options are to use female prosthetics. These are silicon moulds that have a cavity for your male bits but are fashioned on the outside to look like a pussy. The more detailed ones have labia detail, openings, and a cavity like a vagina. The simplest and possibly cheapest is a gaff with a mould like a man's cup but girl shaped. The cup can have definition on the front like lady parts, so it looks more natural through panties or tight trousers. Crossdressing control pants or foundation wear also come made of silicon or similar material in flesh tones and moulded to have female genitals. You wear them like longer shorts but they look like skin. A full body suit may incorporate a bust too. Wear your girl clothes over for a natural look. Downside is they can be expensive. And, obviously, not for everyone.

Shopping List

Okay time for the next shopping list:

Butt pads or lifting panties to make a designer bottom
Tape if you haven't got some already (see last chapter)
Adhesive wound bandages (clear or opaque). A 10cm wide roll can be cut to size.
Gaff or smaller tighter panties (nude skin tone). Get a couple.
Larger pretty panties (cotton or lace) for everyday wear, buy enough for a daily change
Smaller panties for playtime, special occasions, or to wear with certain outfits

A girl can never have too many panties, so this is just a basic starter set. Most items are in the cheaper end of the scale. Day-to-day panties can be bought cheaply in packs. Lingerie style panties can be more expensive because of all the detail, ruffles, and lace. Butt lifters in the 10-20 dollar/pound range. Look on amazon and ebay for the best deals. Ones from crossdressing specific shops can be more expensive but the panties might be more sheer.

Although you can do quite a lot to hide your male bits they still take up some space. As a result, you may find that the panties you choose based on hip or waist size are still a little tight especially around the top of the leg and the crotch area. A tighter pantie can be wonderful for showing off your pretty pussy bump and will hold your tuck more firmly but too tight and the illusion will be spoiled. If you want to be comfortable try panties a size or two up from your hip measurements and also check the gusset area to see if it has extra material to cover a tuck. The latter is usually the case because females need the support for panty liners and so forth but lingerie style and skimpy panties won't have much.

If you cannot dress full time you can still wear nice panties under your man clothes. Don't go too over the top though. Nice cotton panties with some girly detail like a pattern on the front or pretty legs and waist band edging perhaps or with a little bow are fine. Be aware that your shirt might ride up or the top of your panties might be visible over your trousers when you are bending and stretching so a lacy thong or something very feminine is a bit of risk. If you wear the more lingerie style (see next chapter) then you won't be comfortable with your junk and the T-shape of a thong or G-string will raise eyebrows.

Photoshoots and modelling

At the start of the chapter we said you would have that lovely shape that we see in female photoshoots. Clearly if you shape the bottom and tuck your figure will look divine in clothes like pencil skirts and body contoured outfits. But we also promised that special Y shape you see in underwear and swimwear catalogues. That too is possible with a gaff and some tucking even with quite skimpy panties and bikinis.

There is one final set of poses that you may still be intrigued about. These are the glamour shots of Tgirl centrefolds. In these poses the girls wear very revealing lingerie and have curves to die for. Everything looks natural and there is no sign of any taping or other aids. How do they do it?

Well, a lot of the modelling Tgirls are quite far along with hormone treatment so they have true feminine curves because the body has redistributed the fat layers under the skin. A Tgirl on hormones for 1-2yrs will have effects on the genitalia which may make them smaller. In addition to breast implants some girls also opt for castration, this removes the major source of testosterone but also empties the ball sac. Testicle removal takes away the need to pocket and so allows freer movement but can also add curviness as well as making the downstairs area more femme. All this makes it easier to tuck. The empty scrotum may also shrink or can be tightened surgically or removed completely. That gives an overall cleaner profile between the legs.

Remember also that in these modelling shots the models are posing. This means that they can adjust the tuck from shot to shot. In a front shot the tuck is a fold between the legs. In a back or bottom shot the tuck is forward. In a more open leg shot a hand can be discreetly placed so that it looks like it is cupping a pussy not a dicklet. In an all fours shot, the hand can be used to cup and pull the bits forward. In a side view, things are easily hidden. Done well, you'll be hard pushed to spot that she is a Tgirl at all.

We mention this only because if you decide on a makeover with a photoshoot, and are up for it, there might be some lingerie and bedroom shots. It is as well to know what to do with your hands and other bits. And, anyhow it can be fun practicing to be a playboy model in front of your bedroom mirror.

And finally ...

So that's your back and front bits. Now your overall profile is complete. In the next part of the book we will start to build on that foundation.

What you take from these last three chapters depends on your look and what you want to do with girl time. If you are interested only in socialising and enjoying dressing all these techniques will help with your look. If you want a more intimate time, padding, tucking, foundation wear and the other things here will not be that helpful. The emphasis will be more on choosing the right style of bras and panties and other things so you can look the part in the bedroom.

If your aim is to be passable then ensuring that all your curves are in proportion and making sure that front and back aren't obviously fake are the things to go for. However, dressing and feeling feminine are two different things. Sometimes you'll just want to tuck things out of the way so that they don't remind you of maleness. You might find foundation wear too onerous and restricted even though it gives you a better look. Likewise, with breast forms and other forms of chest enhancement.

Only you know the precise combination of things that will make you feel comfortable with your inner female. Go with what works for you. Remember that men and women have similar body types so if you want to feel happy in your skin without enhancements the next part of the book will show you how fabrics and cuts of clothing can add to your femininity. We will also look a little at deportment and posture so you can carry your femme look to the next level

Part 3
Dressing for Success

She was a long cool woman in a black dress
Just a 5'9" beautiful 'n' tall
Just one look I was a bad mess
'Cause that long cool woman had it all

The Hollies (woman in a black dress)

Chapter 7 Lingerie, Stockings and Pretty things

A selection of sexy lingerie should be part of every femme wardrobe. In this chapter we want to cover the basics and weigh up the pros and cons. This is also the last item you will need before you can move onto the other aspects of feminizing yourself with outer clothing, make up, and hair. If you are happy with your work-a-day underwear than skip onto the next chapter. If you want a little more sensuality and sophistication read on.

The word lingerie is taken from the French language meaning undergarments, particularly lightweight items close to the skin. In English it has come to be identified exclusively with intimate underwear, sleepwear, or bedroom items which are extra pretty, cute and/or sexually alluring. Such items are considered especially feminine because they are made of soft and delicate materials. Traditional colours include black, nude, and white but reds, pinks, purples and soft pastels are also popular. There are so many choices that we will only be able to give you a flavour of what is out there. For a coordinated look match or contrast your lingerie to hair, eye, and nail colour.

Some women dismiss lingerie as frivolous or pandering to male ideas of sexuality but wearing lingerie under your outfits can make you feel extra special and will alter the way you carry or present yourself. The quiet shush of sheer material as your outer and inner garments rub together or the cheekiness of ruffles or frilly details will make you feel more sensual. If you are playful in the bedroom, a babydoll or sexy nightie can be super flirty. It is not just down to the cut of the clothing or the challenge of matching a pretty bra with panties though. The types of material make for a soft feminine experience as they touch skin or contrast with your curves and skin tone.

Typical materials

Lingerie differs from everyday cotton panties and bras by the materials used in manufacture. Typically, this includes fabrics such as satin, silk, cotton-satin, muslin, organza and lace. Let's look briefly at these so we know what we are buying or the feel that we want.

Satin weave has a shiny outside surface and a dull back. The shimmer of the material is due to the prism-like structure of the protein fibre obtained from silkworms which reflects light at different angles giving different colours. There are four threads of weft to one warp yarn which ensures that it reflects more light than other cloth materials like plain or twill weaves. The fibres can be silk, polyester, or nylon. A silk material is one where the primary ingredient is just the silk. If the fibres are mixed with cotton it is referred to as sateen (or cotton-satin). The purer the mix of silk the more you are likely to pay. Apart from lingerie and nightgowns satin also appears in blouses, evening gowns, neckties and scarves.

Muslin (or Malmal) is a plain cotton weave which can be made with different weights of fibres from coarse to delicate. The better quality material gives a fine smooth texture suited to light and airy clothing. Underwear made of this material can give you the 'no-panties' feel which is both sensual and naughty. You can have soft but coarser material for work-a-day vests (camisoles) and lighter material for a looser chemise or more intimate garment.

Chiffon, Organza, and Tulle are silk mixes that provide a net like material that can be soft, wrinkle easily, or be stiffer to give clothes more texture. For example, a typical ballet tutu is very stiff and short but still pretty whereas a romantic tutu is longer and softer and falls gracefully below the knee. In lingerie these materials are used to add decorative frills and ruffles. You might also find them used for petticoats to add more volume and with taffeta or tulle which give an evening dress that crunchy swishy sound.

The ultimate yarn for lingerie is lace. Lace can be made from cotton, silk, or linen and has an open net-like structure. A pretty or floral pattern is often sewn onto the netting for a delicate appearance that is used for edging or the main body of an intimate garment. The sewing can add a variety of textures and looks depending on how it is done. The purest form of lace is so-called needle lace where a needle and thread are used to create the pattern. Often this technique is used in bridal dresses and gowns where it is visible but lace is also used extensively in lingerie where it is hidden. A carefully crafted bridal dress gives a hint of what is to come on the honeymoon night.

There are seven types of lace every girl should know about. Alencon lace originates in France and usually has a floral design on the sheer net background. Guipure lace is a venetian lace with patterns made by close embroidered stitches that make the net seem to disappear. Embroidered lace consists of delicate patterns tightly stitched onto an illusion base (so it looks like applique where different textures are sewn together). Chantilly lace has an outline pattern and lots of detail that covers most of the net. Knit lace lacks a tulle back and so is more flexible for contouring the body. Brocade is a delicate shuttle weave made of coloured silks often with gold or silver threads. Eyelet lace (or Broderie Anglaise) has more texture and is made of cotton with small (oval) holes arranged into floral designs and finished with stitching. The latter was most popular between 1840 and 1880 for women's underclothing and is often seen as the detailing on pretty blouses or tops with frills.

The essentials

After a collection of sexy bra and pantie sets for different occasions there are four main things you should consider for your femme wardrobe.

Slips – a slip is something that you wear between your underclothes and your dress or skirt. A full slip has thin shoulder straps and extends from the breasts down to a fashionable skirt length. A half slip starts at the waist. Slips are normally made of silky material and quite plain. They are intended to smooth out your curves and cover bumps in underwear to help the line of a dress or skirt. A full slip allows to you wear sheer or thin fabric blouses or dresses safe in the knowledge that bras and panties or other underwear will be hidden. Together with stockings, slips can add a silky feminine rustle to your movements as they move (or slip) over your figure. In the directoire style they can be used over your foundation wear.

You'll see a lot of slips in movies from the sixties where risqué or intimate scenes have the wife or femme fatale without a dress but in a slip and not showing but hinting at more. A slip can give you a professional, lady boss, or strict look and lends itself to a more mature, sophisticated persona. For example, Elizabeth Taylor in the brooding film *Cat on a hot tin roof*, Anne Bancroft in the *Graduate*, or Betty Draper in the series the *Mad Men*.

Corsets – a corset is a fashionable type of girdle so it can be used as shapewear or as a sexy accessory. Although much reviled in the past a good fitting corset can give you not only curves but improve your self-esteem and confidence as a woman. Corsets can also be made of PVC or leather and be decorated in various ways. If you are into the goth scene, steampunk, or burlesque then a corset is a must. Satin ones are the usual choice if all you want is an hourglass figure because it gives a smoother line. Leather ones can be worn over clothing but tend to stretch after a time. To avoid perspiration and staining of the corset it is best to wear a very thin chemise or other garment underneath. Hence the sexy Victorian boudoir look.

There are several different types of corset to consider. Over the boob ones start just under your armpits. Under the boob ones start just under the breasts. The under bust ones obviously offer no support for your breasts or breast forms so you will need something extra for that. A longline corset extends over the hips (not just the waist) and is good if you have a long torso. A cincher is longer at the front and back but shorter at the sides usually cut in an elegant curve to fit over the hips. A waspie is a smaller cincher like a wider belt and goes around your waist to pull it in (like a wasp body). A Bodice style circles the natural waist area and can have shoulder straps to give support for the whole back and waist. These are useful for shorter torsos and can make your boobs look bigger.

The over bust corsets come in two main varieties cupped or lingerie style. Cupped ones are normally padded and give extra support for the bust. Lingerie corsets are more for display and have lots of detail and usually include (detachable) garters so that they can be worn with stockings. A bustier is somewhere in between the two helping to both shape the waist and lift the boobs. Because they really pull in they are usually only for fashion or playtime but are sometimes used in waist training.

It is important to understand the difference between these styles so that you know what you are paying for. A cincher will suck you in to get an hourglass shape and a bustier generally won't be so extreme. Normally there is a front part (called the busk/busque) which can be tightened by adjusting fastenings but there may also be a set of laces at the back. The corset can give lesser or greater curves and some have extra support such as steel or resin boning to help keep things in place. A properly tightened corset can also pull your ribs in, so they taper into the waist and look more female like. The laces need to be the tightest at the middle to give the best shape and support.

Unlike shapewear that is usually plain, corsets can be very fancy. This means that they are more versatile. You can wear them as everyday underwear as bedroom statements or as fashion accessories. In the latter you can get a classy look with the corset over your blouse or dress to give you the dominatrix look. Wonder woman wears an armoured scrolled corset and Zena the warrior princess a leather one if you want a more amazonian look. PVC and leather under boob ones are ideal for this kind of thing but the fancier over boob ones can work too especially if you can manage to show off your shoulders and neck without a blouse for a sweeter look. Other cuts of corset may help with this.

The flat front style is used to squash in the boobs. It can be a squarer peasant style, but also can have some padding so will help with anything you are doing to give your natural endowment a lift. If you are more daring the sweetheart neckline is an evening gown style and can be used with au-natural taping. Don't forget that you can wear these with tailored trousers and jeans too! Usually a nice up-do hairstyle will set off your look to perfection.

Rompers - are one-piece garments that range from a more leotard or teddy kind of look through to the barely any material playsuit. The top half has narrow straps, the waist is often elasticated but much less so than control wear, and the bottom can be a loose or shaped pantie. Both the bust and leg openings are often decorated with a wider lacy finish, but plain and simple ones are also popular to wear under your regular clothes. There is an enormous choice of styles and detailing so you are sure to find something you like.

Think about wearing a romper after you get out of your foundation wear or corset. You can wear them with or without a bra so they are nice to just relax in and enjoy the silky feel or wear more textured material for a fun night in the bedroom. They can also be worn under day clothes if you don't use a corset or want a freer feel. Likewise, to complement a ladies business suit or blouse-pants combination to give the look of no underwear and smooth lines. The top can act like a camisole or upper part of a slip for thinner blouses or as an undervest for more open shirts.

A romper can also be used as a looser garment after you shave the intimate bits or do your pamper routine. Slip one on and curl up in front of the TV to watch a nice movie or while you are doing nails and other femme things. A tighter pant or a teddy style will help with a tuck but usually they are not elasticated enough to hold anything in place by themselves unless you are tiny. You can also go free and easy with a looser lacy leg trim and cami-knicker type of cut.

Babydolls - complete our essentials. The babydoll style is defined by a dress or nightie that is very short. Usually the item has thin shoulder straps or puff sleeves and covers the boobs in a bra or loose style. The skirt part can hang anywhere between the top of the hips and just below the crotch area. The dresses tend to be a little longer (top of thigh) than a nightie but still short to give a tempting possibility of a knicker flash especially if you are not careful with movement and deportment. If you like the style but don't want to expose your knickers use a pair of tighter shorts (gym style) or even control panties with a leg that matches the colour of the dress. Make sure the shorts or whatever are shorter than the dress!

The name Babydoll came from the title of a 1956 movie starring Carroll Baker as a young nymphet. Not to be confused with the more recent character in the film Suckerpunch which has a different Lolita style sailor look. Babydoll nighties were very popular around the 1950-60s as a fuller cut was used for bridal night wear. Modern day ones have much less material, are over skimpy, and do not leave much to the imagination. They are more like rompers or playsuits. The allure of a babydoll is that it hints or flirts with possibilities. That is good for crossdressing where you want to tease and hide various male features.

If we confine ourselves to the fuller lingerie ones a key characteristic is the way it hangs off the boobs to give a sexy pouty appeal. But they can also be worn straight without any boobs which makes them highly suited for intimate crossdressing, relaxation, or roleplaying. The vintage style uses lots of lacy trim, feathers and ribbons with several layers of chiffon which are flattering to any figure and gives various degrees of transparency. Think that sleepover scene with the pink ladies in the movie *Grease*, the dance scene in Austin Powers, *international man of mystery*, or Britt Ekland as Goodnight in the 007 movie *the man with the golden gun*. The short nature makes them ultra-feminine and flirty.

A babydoll usually comes as a set with matching panties. The panties in older versions tended to be of a fuller cut with lacy bottom frills or rumba style. Which is excellent if you are wanting to hide your male bits without tucking but can also be a point of interest in feminization games and hide a lot if you get easily aroused. Likewise, they can complement or cover over other attire such as plastic panties for sissies. The more modern versions have less of a mystique and tend to have very little material for the dress part and skimpy panties. So probably best avoided unless you are naturally female in proportion, are smaller down under, or can find ones with fuller panties. The good news is that this style is popular with plus-size women because it doesn't hug the curves so much. You should be able to find something that fits well and still looks sexy.

If you like the babydoll style you can complement it with a negligee (or peignoir) which is a longer sheer dressing gown designed for use in the boudoir. First introduced in France in the 18th century they mimicked day dresses of the time with much lighter material often with lots of transparent layers, chiffon, ribbons, and lace. A lot of the older pinup style artwork use this style for a bedroom feel (see the work of Gil Elvgren, 1914-80). The negligees of the 1940s to 1970s are now collectible items. If you want some pure feminine spoil buy a negligee and wear it over your babydoll, romper, or other underwear when you pamper yourself, do your makeup, or are deciding what to wear.

Petticoats

A fuller waist slip is called a petticoat. Usually they have lots of layers and detailing which make them very pretty and add volume to a dress or skirt. The layers and the material make a petticoat a little stiff so that the layers rustle against one another. This 'poofiness' is one of the main attractions.

Petticoats are mostly made of chiffon, taffeta, crinoline, nylon or a material called voile. Voile is a lightweight semi-sheer fabric made of cotton or polyester mix. Air between the layers gives more volume so they don't deflate easily and are more comfortable when sitting. The type of material gives a different degree of poof per layer. Organza gives the most but is heavier. Voile is popular because it doesn't rely on the stiffness of the material for poof so you need lots of lovely delicate layers. A typically full petticoat can have anywhere between 2-8 layers of material. If you have a collection of thinner petticoats you can always layer up to get that ideal feel.

Petticoats look best with fuller skirts or dresses so that there is enough material to drape over the layering. Typically, this means a circle or swing skirt or a dress with a higher waist like an empire cut (just under your boobs) but some tight bodice dresses look gorgeous too. The idea is to wear the petticoat around your waist so that it poofs out the skirt but doesn't show beyond the skirt. Generally, the petticoats should be somewhere between 5 and 15cm shorter than your dress. Some modern dresses have a petticoat edge sewn into the bottom to suggest fullness. And the hint of lacy underskirt can be extra girly.

Petticoat styles: You can give yourself a different look by the shape of the petticoat. There are three main styles: A-line, Bell-shaped, and Square. The latter is often used in dancing because it has a huge fluff to the side and gives the partner more access to your front. The material is cut into a square which is then sewn to a waist band so it gives it a bouncier freer look with lots of swish. A bell-shape (or cupcake) style balloons out from the waist like a bell reaching its widest part towards the bottom of the dress. An extra lining of frill towards the bottom gives it the classic bell edge. An A-line style fans out more or less straight from the waist again reaching the widest extent at the bottom. Choose the style that you want depending on the hip definition you need for your look. A bell shape has a more Victorian feel while an A-line is more graceful and suited to long sweeping evening gowns. Note though that the very wide skirts you see in movies like the *King and I or Gone with the wind* use a hooped cage under the skirt for more support. Petticoats replaced them because they were very unwieldy and difficult to manoeuvre.

Fluffing: For a petticoat to look its best it needs constant fluffing. The longer you wear it the more the weight of the dress and the top layers will deflate so it needs to be fluffed up again. The principle of fluffing is like adding volume to your hair. If you have a fancy style the hair will go limp with time. You toss your hair or muss it up to suddenly get more volume and look perkier. You need to do the same with your petticoats so there will be a constant need for adjusting your skirts.

The technical name for adjusting your petticoat is to make frou-frou. This means to rustle your skirts to allow air back in between the layers. Hold the petticoat on both sides and then flounce your hands up and down in a vigorous motion. You can also do this one handed by holding the skirt and swishing it left to right with a sway of the hips. Watch the movie musical *West side story* for some great dance scenes with skirt swishing. The latter works better if your dress is shorter. It's a very girlie think to do, ruching your skirts. The singer Stevie Nicks of Fleetwood Mac fame had this down to an art form. Watch some of her music videos to see how to rustle sensually.

When you hang the petticoat in the wardrobe put it on a hanger and turn it inside out. Don't fold it or put it into drawer that will just ruin it. If you want to hide it a little buy a petticoat bag like a suit or dress over bag which is designed to help the volume. However, no matter what you do it will eventually loose poofiness and that is where you can use several petticoats to build up the volume your heart desires.

Stockings and garter belts-

Another must for every crossdresser's wardrobe are stockings and suspenders. A stocking is simply a longer leg covering from the toe to above the knee. Often a garter (or suspender) belt is used to help hold them up.

Tights (or pantyhose) must be just about the worst invention on the planet. Leaving aside their practicality they do nothing to show off your feminine shape and get in the way when you need to toilet. The argument is that they are not as cumbersome as having to wear a garter belt and that they don't need as much adjustment to keep the stockings seams straight but that misses the point of why stockings are so feminine.

The allure of stockings is that they are made of very sheer fabric that help hide blemishes on the legs while giving some coverage. They are also lightweight so you can carry spares in case the delicate material gets laddered or torn. A seamed stocking has a line running up the back where the material is stitched together and when combined with heeled shoes elongate the calf for a pleasant elegant look. They also give a hint as to what is underneath (aka garters and lingerie) without being too obvious which is the height of feminine sensuality. Today stockings can be made in one piece, without the seam, but you can buy ones with false (or mock) seams to give the same look.

Stockings are prevented from coming loose, sagging, or slipping down the leg in three main ways. Each one gives you a different feel and sense of security or naughtiness. A traditional garter is just an elasticated band which is often very detailed with lace, frills, and ribbon that slips around the top of the leg to hold the stocking. Think bawdy 17th century comedies with lots of pantalettes and feisty leg kicking. They are the least secure as they can slip down the leg but are popular mainly at weddings. A bride might wear one in addition to a more secure method like a garter.

Hold ups (or thigh highs) have a band at the top to grip the leg. Since there is no agreed sizing for the bands, they can be loose or be tight and might leave red marks on your legs. A more traditional approach is the garter belt which fits around the waist and uses the hips to hold up the stockings by attaching an elasticated fastening (or suspender) that clips onto the stocking top. This is the most secure and many would argue the sexiest.

Garter belts come in all sorts of shapes and sizes from tiny lacy material to more substantial waistbands. Usually they fasten at the back like a bra. Alternatively, the suspender (or stay) can be attached directly to a corset or piece of foundation wear or other lingerie item including panties and rompers. They also have a huge variety of lacy designs making them the ultimate undergarment fashion accessory. The sky is the limit and your choice of garter can help set your mood or personality. Below we give you four main choices.

Retro style – this is a more traditional garter belt that fits high on the waist, is tight fitting and looks like a wider belt. Because of the extra material it can help pull in your waist at the same time. And, because it rides high, you'll never have to think about taking it off for any activity and it won't show through more tight-fitting skirts. It comes with a variety of strap arrangements (2-14) some of which we consider below. You might want to wear a slip over it if you are wearing skimpy blouses.

Four strap – these belts are what you probably think about when we mention stockings and suspenders. They are popular because they show the most thigh and are less fiddly to attach to the stockings. You get two straps for each leg. A front and a back one. This means that the straps are barely noticeable under skirts that fit tight on the hip.

Six strap – is a more robust variety popular with burlesque outfits and mistresses. There are three straps for each leg, a front, back, and side. The additional side strap helps to keep your stockings straight so that the stocking seams won't get out of line as easily. Eight strap and upwards have a more dominatrix look.

Wide garters – are just what is implied they are like a small micro or mini skirt but a lot thinner. They fit more over your waist and hips to give a very secure fit that leave space for a cincher on the waist or can be hidden by your skirt. The lower point of attachment for the suspender means that they are almost completely hidden even for tighter hip skirts and dresses.

If you like the idea of stockings and suspenders but don't want the faff of doing them up you can get tights with the pantie part cut into a suspender and garter shape. With the right cut these can look sexy as well. An extension is the body stocking which extends the tights from the pantie upwards to cover the rest of the torso and sometimes the arms. A firmer cut on the panty part of tights can provide some slimming effects or hold padding.

Know your stockings

Apart from their sheer sexiness stockings have all sorts of detail that can be used to express your femininity. The styling on the heel and toes can emphasise your ankles. The tops (or welt) can be given texture and allure with fancy lace finish or cute bows. The main leg material can be patterned in a variety of ways for a pretty or formal look.

Here are a few things to look for when buying your stockings. First is the denier or thickness of the stocking material. The lower the denier the more sheer or transparent the stocking. Higher the denier the more opaque and warmer they are. A higher denier stocking can also hide any leg hair if you forget to shave. If you are looking for the genuine seamed stocking you need to buy fully fashioned ones, everything else is a mock seam. You can tell the difference because there is usually a finishing loop in the top of the stocking. Mock seamed stockings also tend to have less detail on the ankles and toes.

Traditional stockings have more material underfoot where it is more likely to wear by contact with the shoe. Early on this caused a problem on how to fade the thicker material with the more sheer stocking and a variety of fashionable styles have emerged. A Cuban heel has a short rectangle at the base of the heel up to the start of the calf. A point (or French) heel tapers off to a point. Apparently popular in France because it supposedly mimics the Eiffel tower. A Manhattan heel is again a rectangle but with a border and small point or hat on the top. Supposedly this copies the look of buildings on the skyline of Manhattan.

Other details are the shape of the toe which is also made of thicker material. This is especially important when you wear open toed shoes. And, of course, you can get detailing on the side of the ankle or calf such as floral designs or butterflies or bows and ribbons (a process called clocking). So more than most things the type of stockings you wear can say a lot about your sophistication, personality, or indeed femininity. A nicely turned ankle and calf can be an attraction all by itself. A connoisseur will appreciate the detail in your appearance.

Of course, men have all sorts of fetishes about stockings and pantyhose. From the seamed stockinged pencil skirted mistress or lady boss through to the office secretary, flight attendant, various uniforms (nurse, maid etc), or sexy librarian with a demure opaque or knitted look. If you think opaque is geeky or frumpy, think again. The girl band the Saturday's show what is possible in their music video, *Up*. The preppy look also tends to use opaques or pastel colours. Knee length stockings and ankle socks also have their own admirers.

The man's shirt, panties, and ankle sock look also has a huge following. Try this after a shower as you tuck up on the sofa to dry your hair, talk on the phone, paint your nails, or catch a movie. It is also a popular bedroom look in many movies. Cute it up with some hair ribbons, ponytail or pigtails.

Lolita Fashion

A Lolita dress is a baby doll style dress with a high-volume petticoat underneath. Ideally one uses a short skirt (anything to knee length) and or blouse with a crinoline or short petticoat underneath and often opaque tights, over the knee hold-ups or longer stockings. The style developed from Japanese pop culture influenced by Edwardian and Victorian children clothing styles. If you have ever encountered manga or anime comics, movies, or games, you probably know this style already because many of the heroines or damsels in distress are dressed like this. The emphasis is on adorability or cuteness.

There are entire subcultures ranging from goth, sailor, princess (or hime), erotic (ero), all white (shiro), all black (kuro) to steampunk if you want to explore. A related theme is the sissy in crossdressing and feminization games. It is also popular in cosplay so a possible alternative if you are stuck for a fancy-dress party idea. Mainstream versions are the sexy French maid outfit or cosplay Bo-peep.

In sissy play this style is taken to the extreme with the skirt just down to the top of the thighs so that the petticoats are highly visible. Specialist outlets for sissy play do all sorts of tutu and party dresses in this style but they can be expensive. These types of dresses also tend to have high poofiness so it is very difficult to bend, move, or sit without flashing your knickers which are often highly ruffled or rumba style. As a result, you'll constantly need to be adjusting or making frou-frou with your skirts. If you are roleplaying or have a partner or a mistress feminizing you, they can have endless fun disciplining you for not being lady-like with your little dress.

Men's lingerie and other bits

Next, a quick note about other forms of lingerie. Every so often it becomes fashionable to market male lingerie. By and large this is underwear made of the same materials as female lingerie (but mostly silks and satins) with similar cuts. The panties come with extra material for men bits and the tops are cut like trainer bras with no support or cups. Usually there is less frilliness or lace and they are less flattering on the torso. So far, they have failed to catch-on but the market is growing. One may venture that this is because manufacturers have taken away the essential elements of what makes lingerie pretty and alluring.

Anyway, before we dismiss these items entirely, they can be a nice complement when you aren't fully dressed but want to feel feminine. For example, if you want to wear something under your boy clothes without having to strap or tuck. Alternatively, if you are taking a rest from tucking and want to give some air to the male parts without giving up that femme feeling. They can also be useful right after hair-removal to give your bits a softer feel without chafing in tighter fitting or skimpier girl pants.

You can also find male stockings and tights too. This shouldn't surprise us because tights were fashionable for men in the middle ages. Some men aren't into the full crossdressing scenario but do like wearing stockings and pantyhose. If this is your thing then there is no reason why you cannot wear said items under your normal male clothes and enjoy the silky feel. And, no, it doesn't make you gay or necessarily a transvestite.

A male stocking has a slightly different cut to a female one allowing for variations in the shape of the upper leg, thigh, and knee. In fact, because men tend to carry less fat over their limbs a male leg will often look more alluring than a female leg when in stockings and heels. That's ironic but if you don't find what you are looking for in the female hosiery department or the fit isn't right because of your upper leg development have a look at male ones.

Another fashion accessory mainly for sissy play or mistress games is the pouch or sheath. A pouch is a small bag for the male bits which ties behind the scrotum and base of the penis to keep it in place. They can range from super feminine ones with ribbons, silky and lacy detail through to more bondage style in PVC and leather with studs and locks. A sheath is like a sock for your bits but open at both ends with the heel fitting over the ball sac. Again, these can be made of lacy materials and highly decorated with frills and ribbons. If you don't want to tuck, are in chastity, or want to keep the male parts out of mischief, then you can pretty things up with a girly pouch. Just a thought.

Shopping list

Okay, time for out next shopping list.

Slips (full and/or half)
Rompers (plain for every day, frilly for girl time)
Babydoll (nightie for bedtime dressing or fun)
Negligee (to wear over your under things while pampering or dressing)
Bra and pantie sets (matching pairs are so liberating and femme)
Fashion corset (or two) for different looks
Garter belts (plain for everyday and frilly for playtime)
Choice of stockings (choose to match outfits and personality, you can never have too many)
Petticoats (if you are into this the wardrobe won't be big enough)
Male lingerie (for a day off from tucking or strapping)
Optional pouch/sheath (if you don't want to tuck or to disguise a chastity device)

Slips and Rompers tend to come in around 20 (dollars/pounds) again it depends on the material. The more silky and soft things are the more expensive. Babydolls and negligees depend not just on the material but also the detailing and type of lace finishes. A cheaper nylon mix can cost only 10 (dollars/pounds) and a high fashion sexy look from a brand name like Victoria's Secret or Agent Provocateur can easily be over 50. Likewise, with lingerie bra and panty sets. Fashion corsets can start at 30 (dollars/pounds) and go upwards to hundreds. PVC and leather ones start a bit cheaper but fetish ones with lots of busk and strap detail are more expensive.

Garter belts range from a few pounds/dollars up to the 50s or more depending on the width of the belt, the detailing, and number of stays.

Stockings have a huge range. A cheap pair made of nylon can be a few pounds/dollars. A full silk set easily 20-30 and fully fashioned more depending on the type of heel you want or the fashion house. If you know what you are looking at then a pair of stockings can indicate your social status or how much self-esteem you have for yourself. A cheap pair of fishnets is a bit slutty but a fully-fashioned pair with a quality material, heel finish, and other bits looks classy. Modern stockings are stretchy compared to fully fashioned ones and so are more forgiving on man shaped legs. If you want to slim your legs a bit go for the tighter fully fashioned ones. If your legs are more athletic think about getting a pair of male stockings for a better fit.

Men's lingerie tends to still be on the expensive side at least 20-30 dollars/pounds for any form of cut. Even panties are at the bottom of this range. A nylon sheath a few pounds/dollars. Drawstring pouches are similar. The more fetish and bondage style ones get more expensive depending on the detail and design. Note that you will find more girly pink and frilly looking things with male cuts if you search for sissy lingerie.

As we have said before you get what you pay for. Generally, the purer the material, the more detailing and frills, or the more refined the name or manufacturer the more you are going to pay. If you want specific cuts for the male shape these are usually more expensive than equivalent female items. Not always though so it pays to shop around. Girls love shopping. You knew that, right?

And finally ...

Before we move on, here are a few other things to think about. There is a lot of stuff in the shopping list and it is building up with other things so your closet may be bulging. You might be thinking you cannot purchase stuff because your dressing is a secret and you have nowhere to store everything. If you have a spare room, make it into a crossdressing room where you have femme closets and draws and a make-up table. This keeps it away from your male clothes and stuff and you can add a lock to keep it away from prying eyes or visitors. Surprising how many people have a nosey when they go to the bathroom.

If you are stuck for space or you want to hide it from your partner or family think about hiring a locker. Some makeover and crossdressing friendly locations will rent you some space for a small monthly fee. The better ones also give you a space to dress and do makeup before you go out. Alternatively, you can hire a hotel room for a girly weekend and collect your stuff on the way. If you are discreet most places won't have a problem. Obviously the more passable you are the better. Some places are Tgirl/CD friendly and may organise crossdressers only weekends which can include a social programme or spa treatments. If this appeals to you ask around locally or on crossdressing forums.

Getting dressed in lingerie is probably going to be the first step if you sign up for a makeover session. The idea being to get you into the part and then have your makeup, hair, and nails done. This is not just a time for feminization but also for the social aspect of being girly, a chance to gossip and swap details about what you like. So being knowledgeable about all the above, knowing the names and cuts, and properties of materials will help with that. Likewise think about always dressing in lingerie after a bath or while you are choosing your outfit. This allows you to drop into your femme persona.

Last, but not least, always put your panties on over your suspenders not under if you can. The only exception to this is if the stays are attached to shapewear or a garter below your natural pantie line. It sounds obvious but it's a rookie mistake that is easy to make because tights usually go over panties so that they don't get in the front or back crease and that pads for that special time can fit securely. But with suspenders when it comes to a tinkle or something else you won't be able to get your knickers off without half undressing. Getting your panties in a tangle kills the moment. Enough said!

Chapter 8. Dressing, Fashion, and Heels

In this chapter we are interested not so much in the detail of any clothes you might want to wear but how they fit with your body type or figure. Here are three reasons why you should pay attention to how you dress and the clothes you choose.

First off, this book is all about getting the best male to female makeover you can. If you get everything else right and mess up your ensemble you will stick out to any fashion-conscious female. Men of course will use your dress sense as a filter for girlfriend material, friend with benefits, one nighter, slut, high maintenance, and unobtainable. Crossdressing and all that aside, are you a girl that any prospective partner might want to take home or include you as a friend.

Second, the whole fashion industry is based on giving women options to look more like that ideal hourglass shape or at least to make the best of their features. The difference between a well-dressed woman and someone who doesn't care is remarkable. Think Sandra Bullock in Miss Congeniality. Yes, that is a setup movie – Sandra Bullock has good looks, so she's a diamond in the rough. But the geek to princess, blue stocking to barbie, and other ugly duckling tales that recur in books and movies are all about using your assets to the best.

Third, just wearing the right cut of skirt or blouse will make you look slimmer or more feminine. The patterns and embellishment you use along with other accessories can hide certain features or flatter them. We will look at how patterns and cuts can create illusions in the eye of the observer so that they see something different to what is underneath. For example, making you look slimmer or wider, shorter or taller. If you think this is selling something you are not. A bit of subterfuge is par for the course.

And, of course, this is also another part of your femme socialisation. When you look at glossy fashion mags or chat with your girl friends it will be useful to have something to small talk about. Knowing the cut or style of clothes and how an ensemble is put together or being able to suggest alternatives will add to your feminine persona.

Dressing for your Type

Let's start with the ideal shape and work up to the other body types we saw in chapter 4.

Dressing the hourglass: The golden rule with the hourglass is to avoid anything loose that hangs and hides that gorgeous waist. Clearly anything like that will make you look like a rectangle. Your waist is the centre of attention everything should direct the eye towards it, this will make your other curves stand out even more. This means you are looking for figure hugging dresses like body contoured outfits or tailored clothing and deeper (V) necklines. If you wear blouses with skirts or trousers or wider skirt dresses add a belt or a sash around the waist to grab attention and focus.

If you go for looser material it will tend to hang off your boobs and focus attention there. You might think this is a good idea, but it will make you look top heavy, especially if it is very low cut. And, even worse, you may look as though you are pregnant and trying to hide the bump. Hourglasses do tend to have plenty of bust so you need to make sure that what you wear looks as though it is properly supported (not drooping or sagging to the side) and that your cleavage isn't so deep that it looks inappropriate for the occasion. Party time – deep cleavage, formal events - more modest, workplace – keep the puppies indoors or just a hint with a less revealing cut or a tailored blouse or dress.

Wrap style dresses or soft silks will drape over those curves like a dream as will dresses with a banded waist. The trick is to choose softer less textured fabrics so they can hug onto your figure or pinch into the waist. If by chance you think you are too curvy or voluptuous then you can slim down the hourglass by wearing clothes with vertical details such as stripes or pleats. Darker colours will also make you look slimmer. Hence the little black dress every girl should own. Embrace solid single colours and avoid heavily patterned fabrics at all costs.

If you want to add some volume to your hips (with a fuller skirt or dress) then remember to balance it up at the shoulders to maintain the in-out shape of the hourglass and keep the proportions to hip and bust. For example, princess or puff sleeves. But avoid too much embellishment such as bows or other decorative features at the hip or waist. Also avoid frills and things lower down or up on your bust line which will pull the focus off your waist or make you look wider and lose that proportionality we've worked so hard to get.

Dressing the Pear: We mentioned that the pear shape is one of the more difficult to feminize because it requires adding size to the shoulders. And, that is the trick. Wear anything that will add to your shoulder width or bust area and focus attention on your upper body and away from your lower half. For example, choose a top or dress with a decorative frill over the bust line or that has a shaped shoulder like a puff sleeve, princess, power shoulder pads or other detailing. Choose a bra that will help define and enhance your bust such as a push up or use a little more padding than normal.

Another approach is to wear something extra on top like a cardigan or a looser shirt or maybe even a thick cut jumper. If you think that sounds frumpy, a cardigan with some shoulder detail over a T-shirt complemented with a swing skirt or A-line will look super cute. Think Olivia Newton John as nice Sandy in *Grease*. Alternatively, a top that has hoops. Lighter coloured hoops will make you look wider there which will balance your hips. Layering up on top with a T-shirt and baggy over shirt and things like that are always good to give your upper half a more triangular shape.

To keep the attention away from your bigger hips, avoid pants, tights, or stockings that make your legs look narrow. For example, straight-legged jeans will make your bottom half look like a triangle with the base at your hips. Use normal bottom trousers with heels if possible. Flares can make you look bow-legged. A wider cut or dresses with volume like an A-line also make your hips look more in proportion especially if they hang a little lower off the bottom.

Another trick is to use colour to slim down your hips. Darker colours always have a thinning effect so wear a lighter colour top and a darker skirt on the bottom. A few shades is all that it takes. For example, a white T-shirt with a grey skirt or a lighter pink top with a neutral bottom. If you also add pleats to the skirt that will have a further slimming effect because verticals make you look taller and thinner.

Another illusion is to make people think that it is the cut of the clothing not you that are making the curves. For example, a thin strappy dress on the shoulders with an A-line skirt on the bottom. This is definitely a pear shape but it's the style of the dress. Get it?

Another idea is a strapless dress to show off your shoulders and upper chest with frills and decoration on the top and neutral colours on the bottom. This makes your upper half look more triangular or strawberry. Likewise, a halter neck top or sleeveless square neck dress which has the effect of making you look wider. Remember that what we are doing is balancing up the wider hips at the bottom. A necklace or other detail will also pull eyes upwards. Three quarter sleeves and shirts with wide collars will also work by making you look wider at the top and putting attention on your waist not your hips.

Skirts though must not be tight on the lower body or legs as this will emphasise the hips. Also be aware that some patterns on tights or stockings and lighter pastels will bring attention and make you look shorter. Choose something with lots of details (bows, frills, beads) on the top along with bright colours and patterns. Leave darker slimming shades and plainer materials for the bottom. If you can find dresses and blouses with details on the neck like bows or shaped collars with lace or frills.

Dressing the Apple: Next up is the apple shape. Remember that this shape has a rounder midriff. If you are having troubling pulling it in with shapewear or you get some extra rolls as a result, try some of these ideas. If you find a good combination you can back off the pull-in on the waist and be more comfortable.

Kryptonite for apples is anything that highlights the actual waist. So no thick belts or figure hugging contour dresses or anything that is tight or has a pattern or detail in that area. The emphasis is to pull attention away from your middle to your bust, legs, or arms. All this creates the illusion of a smaller waist.

The first solution to this is to focus attention away from your waist onto the upper and lower thirds of your body. You do this by keeping the details or embellishments on any clothing confined to these areas. For example, by wearing shirts, blouses, and dresses with shoulder details and only slight or limited V-neck lines which will draw attention to your neck. If you have a bigger bust and more cleavage then a V-neck, scalloped or scooped neckline will put attention on your bust and make you look taller but you want to do that without appearing top heavy. That will just make you look dumpy because the weight will be close to your middle.

Also try long-sleeved items that will make your arms look a little bigger but avoid wider cuffs or bell sleeves that will bring attention back to your middle. Alternatively use looser fitting garments on top that will help hide curves you don't want to show. If you want to wear trousers or pants then make sure that they fit low on the hip so that band is lower and doesn't pinch the waist. The same is true for skirts. Heavier fabrics will also wrap around your figure and help anything you are doing to make an hourglass. A weighted fabric will hang straighter and that will make you look slimmer and highlight the shape of your legs. Likewise, embellishments such as bows or sequins will add weight and some flare as well as looking feminine and girly.

It goes without saying that you want to avoid belts or clothes that pinch the waist and so show up your problem area or make you look more solid. Again, a darker plainer colour in this region can have that slimming effect. So colour and frills on top, plain middle, and then further patterning on the bottom half of your dress.

You can also use a great little technique called colour blocking. This means that you mix light and dark colours all the way up and down your body. For example, use a lighter colour down your middle and a darker colour (like black) at the sides. This will give the illusion of shrinking your waist and that your body is more hourglass than it is. It works because our visual system uses darker colours as an indication of curvature or depth. We used this trick previously to create the impression of a cleavage on a flat chest now we are doing it with fabric on your sides.

Higher waist dresses are perfect for apples. Choose a style that has slim belt or tie that lies in the smallest part of your waist towards your bust. For example, an empire line. This moves your waist up a little and the skirt flows over your actual waist. You can do this with narrow bodice dresses too allowing the skirt to hide the apple part of your torso. The bodice will make your upper body appear more triangular and closer to the hourglass. Works even better with a balconette style of bra or a plunging V neckline.

Another trick is to use shorter skirts and dresses. This will expose more of your legs and so pull attention away from your waist area. We talked about sissy dresses in the last section and if you think about what we are describing here it is a short dress that starts just under the bust. That's a babydoll or a tutu dress with the waist hidden by petticoats. No wonder that is a look for sissy males which tend to be more mature in years and have the classic apple shape. The female fashion equivalent is a little more discreet with a longer skirt like a romantic tulle but you get the point.

Dressing the Banana: The straight up and down look or rectangle is more boyish. The idea is to either use clothes that flatter your flapper style body or suggest curves where there aren't any. The obvious solution is to use some sort of corset either under or over your clothes. But when you don't want to do that add a belt or wear a dress that has a sash or built in belt to pinch in the middle. Silky or straight up and down dresses will also work at an evening event such as dance or dinner. Empire line dresses and simple shift dresses suit your body type but can look a little plain and frumpy. Especially if your tummy isn't that flat. Choose ones that have a bit of shape in them.

To build up the bust area think about adding extra padding or a cup size to your bra or breast forms especially if they look a little lost on your chest. Lots of texture like frills and ruffles will give your bust more apparent volume. And with something like an off-the-shoulder gypsy top finished with broderie anglaise you can make your shoulders look wider. Sleeveless dresses will also make the best of your lean arms. Together this will give the illusion of a triangle into your waist. Likewise, if you choose a dress with embellishments like bows or brocade or brooches or scoops on the bust area or neck.

In the lower half you probably have reasonable length legs that are not too skinny or wide. Make the most of this by showing them off with miniskirts and dresses about the knee. Because mini's are usually tighter fitting they will put emphasis on your butt and hug onto your legs which will make you look more hippy. Likewise, for shorter skater and tutu like dresses with an A-line, you'll make a triangle into your waist. Choose dresses and skirts that have volume or layers such as a classic tassel flapper dress.

The thing to avoid is looking too boyish. You probably will look good in jeans and t-shirt or sweatpants or gym stuff. But your smaller than average sized bust puts you in the tom-boy category. If you do want to be in the gym, wear figure hugging stuff designed for female workouts (which is a bit like shapewear) to give you some curves. Avoid shapeless dresses and high necklines such as boat neck cuts that will make you look taller, skinnier, and more oblong. If do want to wear jeans or trousers then don't choose baggy or saggy ones. A tight fit will give you hips and butt.

Dressing the strawberry: The strawberry is the female version of tarzan (or type 1) with an inverted triangle shape wide at the shoulders and narrowest at the hips. A Rhomboid is a common variation in which you have a bit of waist which cuts off the end of the triangle. Given what we have noticed above, dressing for this type is really easy. You want to draw in your shoulders, emphasise your middle, and flare out your lower half to give a sense of hippiness.

Choose darker unfussy tops with less detail or embellishment. Add some neckline like a V shape that will pull your eyes away from your shoulder and down to your bust area which is narrower. Recall that on average the width of male shoulders is 2.5 heads whereas a female it is more like two heads. So plain sleeves that are darker or solid colour and a lighter colour on the chest area will chop off that extra 0.5.

Make the most of your waist area with a belt or a little detail. The latter might make you look a little wider but it will make your shoulders look less out there. You can also add long sleeves with some detail on the cuffs or flared sleeves on the lower half again to pull the eye downwards.

For the lower half the thing is flared skirts or dresses. Anything that makes you look hippy and builds volume outwards to match your shoulders will make you appear more hourglass. The watch words are swish and volume. A dress or skirt that moves around you is not only feminine but distracts the eye. A-lines and Bells with petticoats give you hips. And patterns and pretty embellishments with brighter colours will again give you a counterbalance to wider shoulders. This also tends to limit the length of skirt because it is difficult to get the width without length. For example, a full length A-line evening gown, compared to a knee length bell or cupcake shape, versus a shorter or more tutu look. The more distance between the shoulders and the widest part of the dress/skirt the more hourglass the line and the less noticeable your shoulders are.

Things to avoid are clothes or cuts that emphasise your upper body triangle. Boat necklines or Chinese collars will bring the eye to your shoulder width. A bodice style dress is not out of the question but make sure the bottom (skirt) half is wider than your shoulders. With the right skirt you might also be able to carry off a small puff sleeve or a thinner strapped dress. Of course, tight skirts that hug the hips and legs are a no-no. They just make that upper triangle more apparent and more dominatrix style. If you do want to wear a contoured dress try one with a little looseness or use colour blocking with the lighter colours on the hips and the darker colours on the middle. This will have the illusion of pushing your hips out.

The long or short of dressing

Another way to look at your body is your skeletal or bone structure, muscle, and predisposition for depositing fat in certain places that adds to your shape. In chapter 2 we defined the three types ectomorph, endomorph, and mesomorph. Ectos are lean, up and down, and usually tall. Endos carry more weight being wider and shorter making them look curvier and stocky. Mesos are like goldilocks not too tall and not too short, not too wide and not too thin. Muscular development and bone structure also explain why your arms and legs are longer or shorter or look chunkier or thin.

We've seen some recurrent tips in the examples above. To make your curves more obvious the idea is to use lighter colours and things with flare, embellishment or detail. Printed and patterned material will give you volume. Fabrics with a bit of shine such as satin or pvc will give some further pop. If you are not as curvy as you want to be you can bring out what you have with skirts that taper into your waist and fit snug on the thighs. The obvious example is the pencil skirt which always gives the illusion of curves.

To take attention away from curves we use dark colours and vertical details or embellishments like stripes, pleats, and darts. This will not only narrow and elongate your body but with the solid colours like black, burgundy, navy blue, and olive greens will have an extra slimming effect. If you are too hippy or earth mother draw attention away from that area with details or accessories on the upper half of your body. For example, a necklace or flowers, a brooch or ribbon. And to hide the waist or hips use flared skirt materials with fuller skirts. If your thighs are the problem then use a fit and flare skirt which comes down over your hips before the skirt flares out to hide the thighs.

Heavier fabrics that have some weight and resistance will help slim and trim your figure. For example, denim, leather, and some linens. A leather skirt with a decent waist band can pull in your tummy. If you are a muffin-top with bits falling over your waistline, skirts with higher waist band will help control anything that rolls or hangs. A skirt or dress with flounce or flare doesn't just affect your sides. It will also help disguise a front or tummy bulge. This is why higher waisted skirts with flare or empire style dresses are so good for apples.

You can make your legs look longer by raising the hemline of your skirt or dress. Anything above the knee will make you look slimmer and taller provided the rest of the leg is plain or simple. Use less patterned stockings or tights and pastel colours or nudes. Opaques with solid colours only work if your legs are slim otherwise they will add chunkiness. The elongation effect can be developed further if you match your skirt colours to your skin, stocking, or shoe colours. If your skirt or dress is patterned or printed match your stockings and shoes to only one colour.

If your legs are a bit chunky lower the hemline to knee. This will hide any athletic look on the upper legs. You can still wear tight or hip hugging clothes just bring the hem down so that it sculpts the curves. Don't make the material too tight though as this will just define your legs more rather than the thigh. If you have wider calves bring the hemline down further but make sure it falls either just above or just below your calves. If it rests in the middle that will just make the calf look wider. Hobble skirts are great for this. But if you are worried about bigger hips use something like a trumpet skirt or a mermaid dress which hugs the upper legs but then flares out at the bottom.

Another trick that works for all leg types are heels. Heels give you height. Your legs look proportionally longer and you are taller which translates to slimmer in the minds eye. In addition. you also arch or point your foot and this pulls the tendons in your ankle which stretches the calf muscle making it longer and slimmer. This is so important to the femme look that we will be devoting more time to it later.

More on Skirts

You should be getting the picture now that the skirt (including the skirt part of a dress) is of enormous importance in getting your look right. There are at least fourteen basic types of skirt and an almost endless variety of names that go with fads and fashions. We've mentioned a lot of types of skirt already so it might be useful to give you a little A-Z.

Basic types:

A *flared skirt* is anything that has volume at the waist and falls away over the hips. They can be patterned or cut in a variety of ways. The basic cuts are *A-line* (like the letter A), *Bell shaped* (as we saw in the last chapter), and *Circle*. The circle skirt is cut into sections to make a circle at the waist this means it is very full and hangs smoothly without need of shaping with darts or pleats or gathering at the waist.

The next three types are *Divided, Full,* and *Gored skirts*. A divided skirt looks like a skirt but has legs like shorts. They are usually called culottes but a more modern name is skort. Culottes tend to be longer and skorts are short like gym class. A full skirt is like a circle skirt but the fullness is gathered at the waist to give some vertical folds. A gored skirt is one that fits and drops away from the waistline before it flares (sometimes called fit and flare). Usually they are made in sections (anything from four to twenty-four) so that it has some vertical definition.

The next three are *pleated, straight,* and *wraparound*. A pleated skirt has fullness but this is reduced to fit the waist by pleats in the material.

Material is folded vertically and then joined to the waist band. An inverted pleat brings two folds of fabric to a centre line in the front and back so that the sides are straight. This gives smooth hips and a little inverted V on the front or back for freer movement. A straight skirt is a tailored skirt which uses darts to curve the material over the hips. The most obvious example is the pencil skirt. Sometimes a pleat (called a kick) is added at the hem to give a little more leg movement. The wrapround skirt does what it says, it wraps around the waist with the material overlapping on one side and pinned or belted. In dress form this is a very elegant look reminiscent of Greek goddesses and can be of heavier or light material. Gorgeous with curvy hourglasses.

The tenth item on our list is the *underskirt*. This a plain or simple skirt designed for other material or overskirt to hang over the top. We saw some of these in the last chapter. Petticoats and slips are examples.

Basic lengths:

The next four types are all to do with the length. We have *short (micro, mini)* and *long (midi, maxi)*. A short skirt is anything with a hemline that is above your knee and a long one is below the knee.

Typically, a maxi is loose and flowing and extends down to the ankles. Ball gowns are examples. A midi ends at mid-calf and can make you look shorter and wider. Midi's look better with heels and if you are shorter a smaller size will flatter more because of the cut.

A mini is a skirt with the hemline at mid-thigh (usually not more than 4" (10cm) from the knee). A micro skirt is even shorter and ends just under the buttocks. Dresses are mini, micro, midi, or maxi depending on the length of skirt they have.

Fads and fashion:

Of course, all the above types can be combined to get different looks that come in and out of fashion. Here are twelve types that you might see when you're shopping. Some are for every day, some are for clubbing or nightlife, and some are more peculiar.

A cargo skirt is an everyday kind of skirt that often has pockets and belt hoops. They are based on the military style cargo pants and can come in khaki or camouflage as well as other colours.

A denim (or jeans) skirt is highly popular and is based on the 5-pocket jean style. It tends to be shorter like a mini pencil skirt but may have a zip or button up on the front. Sometimes it can have a pinafore top to extend it into a cute girl-next-door dungaree kind of dress.

A *T-skirt* is a skirt that is made from a recycled T-shirt. They often fit like pencil or denim skirts. If you are handy with a needle and thread, make your own.

A *skater skirt* is a short high-waisted circle skirt that is made of light material so that it swings like an ice skaters costume. The hemline is usually above the knee. A variant is the baby doll dress where the skirt is often fuller and the hem is more a mini or micro length.

A *bubble (tulip or balloon) skirt* has a lot of volume that puffs out like a balloon and then has the hem tucked back underneath to form a kind of bubble.

A *bouffant (or puffball) skirt* is similar to the bubble except that the hem doesn't tuck under it just comes to a natural tighter circle around the legs. This gives it the puffy silhouette but restricts movement.

A *swing skirt* is a flared or circle skirt that is fitted on the hips with pleats and darts and a wide flare at the hem. Very popular for dancing and other activities where swishiness is the key.

A *wiggle skirt (or dress)* in contrast is a tight skirt that has the hemline so small that it restricts leg movement. Hence the name. The effect is to make your hips sway more as you walk with smaller steps. Tighter dresses that fall around the calves also tend to have this property for example the trumpet, mermaid or hobble skirt. The body contour dress is a shorter version which is tight on the thigh.

A *tiered skirt* (or dress) is one that has series of separate layers usually getting wider as they go towards the hem. A tassel dress is one form and a Rah-Rah skirt is another. They have a nice girly look and swish without being too formal.

A *crinoline* is a full skirt with a cage or hoop to support the weight along with lots of petticoats (think southern belle). The modern equivalent is a mini-crini which is a short version above the knees but with a lot of outward support.

A *ballerina skirt* is a midi skirt which drops to about mid-calf but has a full voluminous style. When combined with a bodice to make a dress you get the classic 1950s housewife look. A modern version is made of Tulle or Chiffon for a wispy romantic look. A mini or micro version is a tutu.

A *Dirndl skirt* is made of a straight length of fabric and gathered at the waist to give volume. Think Sound of Music or Austrian peasant. In dress form the full skirt has a tight bodice and buxom chest line. A complement is an apron or pinafore. The style is easily modified to a mini or micro form for a sexy milkmaid look or sissy play.

Keeping it demure

Women show much more of their bodies when they dress than men whether this is a sleeveless top, a cut that shows off the cleavage, or an above the knee skirt or dress. The fabrics and materials might also be sheer or thin so that if you are not careful you might show more than you imagined.

Here are several things to watch out for.

Micro vs mini: First, of course, is the micro versus mini debate. Young women today love to show their legs and the short body contoured mini dress is a staple for the nightclub. Micro skirts though are often confined to porn or gentleman's clubs. If you do want to wear one out at party or for fun make sure you wear sensible panties with some coverage. Unless you are an expert tucker, you are likely to give more away than you bargained for. A mini dress is much easier to carry off. You can often wear above knee skirts in the office. It's okay for a secretarial position but the more professional roles require more modest (knee or lower) skirts. A few years back a report leaked from a blue-chip firm caused much mirth and laughter with dress guidelines that advised female staff that a skirt should be no more than a pen length above the knee.

Thin or sheer: If the material of your outfit is very sheer or thin then you need to think about wearing a slip. This includes skirts/dresses that are made of light materials like tulle, chiffon, thin cotton, or have a lacy pattern. If you can see your legs through your skirt or body through the pattern you should also wear a slip. Choose a slip colour that matches or complements your skirt or dress. And, if you do want to give a hint of something more choose a slip colour that matches your skin tone. This is still teasy but much nicer and more lady-like than showing your underwear or whatever.

Tight or Fitted: If your outfit is very tight or fitted and you are not going commando (or knickerless) you need to have seamless underwear. Ideally you need things without side seams or elastic in the leg that can grip your butt and make a groove for the tight material to fit into. If you can, wear a thong or a G-string, if not something with an open leg or lacy finish. Likewise, choose a bra with very little underwiring in the cup or seams in the band. You can get these from, guess where, a good lingerie store.

Visible underwear: Finally, and it might seem obvious, wear skin-toned underwear under light coloured skirts. Most people think if you are wearing something like a white skirt or dress you should wear white bra and panties. But, guess what, this will actually make your underwear more visible. Think about it, lighter thinner material will show your skin tone through. Your knickers just make the material look thicker and so you get a profile of your intimates. Make sure you buy panties and what-not that are close to you own skin tone. So-called nude coloured underwear is just a shade of beige and may not match your natural tone. For example, if you have a pale skin look for ivory or cream. If you are darker use a brown or black. If you are struggling to find these items, then again, a good quality lingerie outlet will have something.

Types of Heels

This next section is all about shoes. In particular that quintessential feminine look of heels. It can't be said that you are a fully signed up crossdresser until you have learned to walk in heels. The next chapter is devoted to how to carry yourself and walk but before that let's see what kind of things are available.

Like skirts heeled shoes come in a number of makes and then there are an unlimited number of variations and styles that can be used to complement your look. Here is the top ten that every girl should know about.

Pumps: are shoes that are low cut on the front to reveal the top (arch) of your foot and tend to be wider than most other shoes. They are the most comfortable and common fashion shoe and can come with no heel all the way up to about 4 inches. A small heeled version (2 in) is often called a court shoe reputedly because ladies of the royal court used to wear them. They make good everyday shoes and are an effective starter for learning to walk in higher heels.

Stilettos (or spikes): take their name from a narrow dagger so the heel is higher and thinner coming to its narrowest where the heel touches the ground. These are the ones that you are likely to see if a girl is wearing mid to higher heels. They start at 1 inch but go up to 10 inches. Because the higher heels tend to arch your foot quite a lot, they are difficult to master. Which is why they are regarded as the ultimate feminine shoe.

Wedges: are an in between type of shoe in that they have the lift of the heel but the gap between the ball of the foot and heel is filled in with a wedge of material. The filling means they distribute your weight more evenly over the foot rather than through the toes like a stiletto. This makes them easier and more comfortable to walk in. They make a good training shoe to master walking in higher heels.

Platforms: are shoes that have extra thickness under the sole. They are a good alternative if you want more heel height but are not so good at balancing. If you think about it there is only so far that your foot can arch into that tippy toe position. The length of your foot will dictate what height of heel you can manage. You often see shorter women using platforms because their feet are smaller and their ability to take a straight high heel is limited. With a platform you can add the extra height you want with the thickness of the sole. For example, if you can walk well in 3 in heels you can bump that up to six inches with a 3in platform.

Cones: are shoes with heels which look like ice cream cones. The wide part is at the top and the smallest at the bottom of the heel. They are like stilettos but wider on the base and chunkier on the top for more support. Like most styles they come in different heights and are still challenging to walk in but not as much as a narrower stiletto because the downward pressure is distributed in the wider heel base making it easier to balance.

Kittens: these heels are still cone shaped, but the height of the heel is restricted to one or two inches. They are a very popular shoe because they give you some lift but are easy to walk in. Because the pressure on your toes and ball of your foot are much less you can stay on your feet longer. Thus, they are good for work shoes or shopping or parties. Most people can master walking in kitten heels in a few minutes.

The next five types of shoe are not so much about the heel but the design of the upper part covering your foot.

Ankle straps: in this shoe you get extra support to keep the shoe in place with a small strap around your ankle. The strap normally attaches to the heel but can also join to the front of the shoe. If you wore T-bar shoes when you were little you'll have the idea except that adult equivalents are way more stylish. Use this shoe if you need to support your weight more when walking.

Peep-Toes: are a bit of a tease because they are cut away on the front so that toes can be seen. They are girly shoes because you need to have a good pedicure and paint your toes for them to look stunning. They come in different heel heights but the higher you go the more your toes get squashed into the hole. Although most women will say wear the highest heel you can to make your toe, heel, ankle, calf combination as elegant as possible.

Cut outs: carry the peep toe idea further by allowing other sections of the shoe to be removed. As well as the top or arch of the foot (like a pump) you can cut out the sides (or arches) or even have an intricate lattice design. Cut-outs are seen as the most stylish shoe because fashion designers can create a unique look by combining the cut-out pattern with the heel height.

Slingbacks: are our last type and designed to help give you support when you walk. Unlike the ankle strap they only have a strap that hooks behind your foot just above the heel. This can stop the shoe slipping forward as you walk but are also easy to slip off when you want to give your feet a rest. A comprise between a comfortable shoe and something more stylish.

As you get into your dressing, you'll find that you have a favourite go-to shoe but try them all. It is often said that a girl can't have too many shoes. In any closet you need a few styles from more modest work heels (like pumps and kittens) to something with a bit more height for parties and going out. You will need multiple types with different fashion design and colours so you can match your wardrobe and set off the rest of your ensemble. If you are on a budget go with neutral colours which can be matched to more outfits.

Finding the right shoes

Make sure you get the right size shoes! It sounds obvious but sizing isn't consistent across manufacturers so you might be a size different depending on the make. If you are a 7-8 male size, you should have no problems finding girl shoes to fit. If you are bigger then look at outsize and plus size shops. And if your feet are really big then crossdressing outlets will have something.

Remember the ideal height for a woman is 5'8". If you are 5'5" then you can easily get away with a 2-3 inch heel. If you are taller or want higher heels then think about your final height. Most women are slightly shorter than a male colleague so anything that takes you over 6' will make you stick out in a crowd. Of course, there are tall women, but they tend to wear flats or low heels like court shoes or kittens. Big heels are also seen as more girly girl than professional. A lot of professional firms will limit the height in the dress code to the 2"-3". So, a demure comprise is a shorter heel with a cut that shows feminine class.

The higher heels are more challenging to walk in and will give you that girly look. Be careful not to push it too far otherwise you'll stop being classy and look trashy. Big heels are often associated with big chested women and the contoured micro-dress. If you haven't got your balance and deportment down, you'll lurch and totter. That can look barbie cute but, on a night out, it can also give the impression that you are tipsy or a little worse for wear. Not something to emulate at the office party.

If at all possible, try your shoes on before you buy. Get a slightly bigger size if they aren't an exact fit. Larger ones might slip off your heel when you walk but that is way better (and a little more femme) than crushing your toes as they push down onto the ball. Also, your feet change as you get older. Gravity pulls your foot out and your arches down so if you haven't worn a pair of shoes for a while you might find they are tighter than you expect. And, of course this means you will have to restock every now and then.

Breaking in your heels is essential if you are to avoid blisters, sore ankles, heels, and toes as well as embarrassing yourself by going arse over tit. Stretching the fabric will help with the former and leaving balance aside the latter will depend on the surface walked on. Polished wood or tiles (like dance floors) are the worst. Most heels have zero grip. Make sure you scuff up the underside of the shoe so there is a bit more friction when you walk.

Finding your colours

We can't leave this chapter without a little advice on how to mix and match colours. It's not all about shocking pink and tutus no matter what some people might think about crossdressing. Ideally, you want to blend in and be passable. Then you can go about enjoying your femme time without hassle. If you make an effort to fit in people will accommodate. So, in these last few paragraphs here are some tips on making your ensemble work.

Colour profile: First up is finding your colour profile. For this you need to know not just your skin tone but also your skin's undertone. The easiest way to do this is to get a piece of silver and a piece of gold jewellery like a bracelet. Slip one onto each wrist and then check them out in a mirror. Which one adds more to your skin and complexion by providing a contrast. If it is gold you should look for warm colours in your outfits. If it is silver, you want cooler colours. If you can't decide then you're probably neutral

A warm colour is anything that has a red, orange or yellowish look. A cool colour has blue, greens, purples and it has to be said some lighter pinks even though pink is a mixture of red and white. Anything else like brown, grey, olive, beige, black etc are all neutrals. Your colour profile is a range over one or two warm, cool, or neutral colours depending on your profile. You can get swatch books with these colours like paint cards for decorating except for fabrics and eye makeup. Get the one that matches your profile and use it to choose the colour of your clothes.

Here is how to get the best combination of colours and clothes:

Match your skin undertone: you will look better in colours that match your undertone and complement your skin tone. This means that you will get a range of colours that work for you. For example, if your skin is pale use richer darker tones of your colours (e.g ruby lips on a white face). Darker skin works better with the brighter tones in your range (e.g. an orange or yellow flower pattern). And if your skin is in between then neutrals will look stunning (e.g. nude nail polish or mauves and beige if you are a brunette with brown eyes and mid to light skin).

Use Neutrals: the next tip is to use accessories and neutrals to complement your main colours. Accessories include shoes, bags, scarves, glasses, hats, gloves, and things for your hair like bands and ribbons. Normally these will come in the neutral colours (gray, black, navy, brown, white, cream) but you can also use a mid-range something in your colour profile for a bit of extra pop. Check which ones work for you. If they make your skin look too yellowy or sickly green or too reddish that colour doesn't work for you.

The idea is to have a mixture of neutral clothes in your wardrobe as well as the accessories. A general principle is that you only choose one neutral per outfit. For example, a coloured dress in your colour range complemented by a neutral like a nice brown belt or a cream blouse with a skirt in your colour profile. Or a more patterned dress with a cream hair ribbon or a black hair band. Get the idea?

Coordinate: The next tip is to coordinate your wardrobe. Choose as many things as you want or can afford from your colour profile and neutrals. The fun is in mixing and matching. Hold them up in front of the mirror to find out what works together. Try one main colour, a neutral colour, and something to pick out the main colour like a slightly different opposite shade from your profile. This way you can choose patterned outfits. Add more than these three colours and your outfit will look cluttered. That will undo any work you have done on dressing for your body type.

Apart from the style and cut of clothes colour says something about your personality. Bright colours tend to be more extrovert and single you out. Light and earthy colours make you look friendly and approachable. Dark and mono colours indicate authority and distance. Hence the business suit look. Paler colours tend to be quieter and more introverted allowing you to blend into the background. Think about this when you are dressing for work, a formal event, or at a party and decide what image you want to project. Are you the life-and-soul of the party, a little wall flower, or somewhere inbetween?

Shopping List

We have covered a lot in this chapter. And, it is not really possible to give you an itemised list. What you buy or add to your wardrobe depends on your look, how much you are going to dress, and your budget. Even if you think you can get away with just a couple of things because your dressing is only occasional, you'll still need stuff. For example, something ordinary and sweet for camming or just enjoying femme time. Then something for day trips shopping or a trip to a club or bar. The more glam and revealing outfits for party time will not cut it if you just want to go window shopping.

A balanced wardrobe will have a mix of skirts and tops, dresses, and heels plus other accessories like jewellery, scarves, glasses, and bags. Skirts and tops are more versatile than dresses because you can mix and match allowing you to have lots of different outfits without too much outlay. Every girl loves a nice dress though, so you'll need something in that line. Your look might dictate the type of dresses you want to wear. Your body type will help choose colours and styling.

If you are roleplaying, your requirements might be very specific but if not don't go for the more exotic things that you'll only wear once in blue moon. You'll want things that you can enjoy regular girl time in and do your everyday stuff around the house. If you do yearn for the more exotic think about a makeover visit where you can rifle through a bigger wardrobe. If you like something there buy one. Often you won't know till you try it on and spend time in it. Your budget is probably too tight to make big mistakes.

We haven't really covered accessories in detail. You can buy and use valuable jewellery and the like if you want to or that has value to you because it is a gift. However, you should think about costume jewellery and cheaper things to accessorize with. Bangles, bracelets, necklaces and so on can distract the eye from your less curvy bits just as effectively as the cut of your dress or skirt. Chunky jewellery can add weight and help to balance your upper and lower halves. Most jewellery goes on the upper torso. So, if you have slimmer hips and need definition use a chunky bracelet. If you want to distract from your waist use a chunky necklace.

Another thing that every girl must have is a little bag. Because you don't have pockets, you'll need somewhere to keep your driving license, phone and money or cards, a place for cosmetics, and of course any materials for tucking and taping just in case. You might also carry some spare stockings in case of a ladder. Maybe even a bit of hand cream or nail file and tissues in case you snag something. Of course, there are as many bag styles as there are shoes or skirts. You'll need a few to mix and match. We're not going to go through them here.

Choose what you like but don't make it too big. One's with detachable straps are wonderfully versatile. You can use them for events or parties without the strap (like a clutch bag or purse). If you get one with a thinner longer strap you can put it over one shoulder and across your chest to the other hip. This is nicely secure and less easy to grab. And, of course, it draws attention to your bust and other curves which is delightfully cute and feminine.

And Finally …

Outfit selection and creating combos that work for you is the fun part of being a girl. Although we have given some guidelines above its up to you to develop your look and find out what works for you. Whenever you are en-femme devote a little time to flipping through the fashion mags or surfing on-line. Look at the styles and the models see what goes with what. Steal an idea or re-purpose one to get your feminine look honed.

If you are brave or comfortable enough or have some girlfriends to go out with have a day shopping. Browse or window shop and if you find something buy it. Nothing more satisfying than coming back from a trip into town with some bags of clothes or a new pair of shoes. Enjoy trying your stuff on and choosing the right accessories and jewellery. Wear your heels.

This way you'll get expert at posing in front of a mirror and that will help your movement and posture.

Waiting rooms are full of women's magazine so if it is a trip to the hair salon, the nail bar, or the beauty parlour for some depilation and pampering you will be able to devote a little time to scanning the latest fashions and fads. You'll also be able to catchup on makeup and hair styles too but that's another story altogether. You can even do this if you are not dressed like at the doctor's surgery, dentist, hotel lobby, or any waiting area.

If you follow the above advice, you'll not only start to feel more girly inside but also know what you want outside. You'll be able to answer all the questions for a makeover and know what you want to try or indulge in that you don't have the budget for at home. You'll also have something to chat about for a few hours, or even be able to pose for some nice photos of the femme you.

Chapter 9. Movement and Posture

This next chapter completes your education into feminizing your body. The difference between the way women walk, sit, and move and the way men do it is one of the biggest tells in crossdressing. We will give you some simple guidelines and advice in the following pages.

An interesting question is to what degree deportment and behaviour is derived from social and cultural conventions or down to the mechanics of movement. We will look briefly at the physics to highlight the differences between male and female anatomy and show that certain ways of moving are more natural for the female frame. You'll need to emulate these to have a convincing look. Of course, one of the biggest topics in this area is to be able to walk and stand properly in heels.

We will also give you a few do's and don'ts. These will add to your increasing female socialisation skills and not only help you feel more feminine inside but allow you to deport yourself in a way that will keep things modest and demure. All this will at least stop you looking ungainly and build a little grace into your movement. How you behave otherwise is entirely up to you.

Centre of Gravity

Our first topic is centre of gravity (cog). Understanding your cog is vital in maintaining your balance and poise. Especially when you are mastering your walk. Some of this is quite technical. Stick with it and you'll end up with a much better outcome.

What is centre of gravity? If you throw a ball straight up into the air it comes straight back down because gravity pulls it towards the ground. The ball behaves like all its mass acts at a single point which is called the centre of gravity. A shape like the ball has the centre of gravity, you guessed it, at the centre of a ball or sphere. We can draw an arrow straight down from the centre of gravity to the ground through the ball which shows how it will fall. The way the mass is moving is also important. If you throw the ball more to the side, it will arch upwards and then down to the ground. The line of action (or attraction) is always straight down through the centre of gravity but the ball moves further away as it drops making the arc. Simple.

Most things including people are not nice neat shapes like balls this means that gravity affects them in more complicated ways. The way your mass is distributed affects the way you will fall when gravity gets a hold of you. Because we are made of muscle, bone, and flesh which have different densities of mass our centre of gravity is not in our centre. If you are not careful, when you move, you can get unbalanced. This happens when the line of action moves outside your base of support.

So where is our centre of gravity? And, yes, it is different for males and females.

Your skull is the heaviest and densest part of your body and accounts for one third of your mass. Likewise, all our organs are in the chest and abdomen. In short this pulls your centre of gravity up into the top half of your body. A man with more muscle development in the upper torso (remember type 1 bodies) has his centre of gravity around the sternum (where the ribs join in the centre of the chest). A woman on the other hand has a bigger pelvis and fatty hips and boobs which counterbalance the head giving a lower centre of gravity just below the navel or top of the pelvis.

Or, measured another way, in females it is located at approximately 55% of the standing height, whereas in males it is approximately 57% from your feet.

Crossdressing and Centre of Gravity

Here are four reasons why your cog is important in crossdressing.

First, when you bend over the extra mass of your breast forms or boobs will swing forward and move your line of action differently to what you expect. You'll have to compensate to how you usually bend and recover to stay balanced. We'll show you how later.

Second, female breast tissue is heavy and without a bra unsupported. There is a little bit of connective tissue that helps stabilise things, but breasts move a lot when women exercise. Biomechanical studies show that when women run (braless) their breasts jiggle up and down and swing side to side by several inches. Imagine those Baywatch babes running along the beach. That's why a woman should always wear a sports bra when she goes to the gym. Walking quickly will also build these side to side movements due to hip motion. If your pace is too fast, you'll get that up down movement as well. Your breast forms or whatever are even less well connected than female boobs. Those oscillations are going to be worse for you than the average female. Below we'll show you how to control boob swing.

Third, when you are in heels, you will be tipped forward. You are effectively on tippy toes. This moves your centre of gravity higher. The tendency is to lean back. This can tip your line of action out through your back. You will have to learn to control your natural movements in a different way because you only have a little platform (the balls of your feet) to counterbalance. If you get this slightly wrong and lurch forward or to the sides the moving mass in the boobs will exaggerate the effect and pull you quickly off balance. The higher your heels the more dramatic this will be because they lift your cog higher which makes you less grounded and more unstable. We'll look at tipping points and how to watch where you walk to avoid problems.

Fourth, but not least. Because the cut of female clothes often restricts movement the obvious or instinctive correction to balance is sometimes not an option. You won't necessarily be able to put your feet, legs, or torso where you want to without being restricted by material or revealing too much. Or, if you do, you won't look very lady-like. The characteristic way women move is related to how they have trained themselves to stay balanced while maintaining modesty and dignity. And, you thought all that preoccupation with ballet and yoga was just because it is was a girly thing to do.

Feminine Posture

To get a realistic female look you need to have boobs that have the same mass as they would be if you were female. A good bra helps give support and spread the load onto the shoulders but you need to do more if you are to avoid long-term back and neck problems.

Here is a simple trick to give you the right alignment. Imagine that there is a thread through the top of your head pulling you upwards and straight. This will push back your shoulders and make your chest (boobs) stick out a little more and pull in your tummy. Don't push them out so far that you have to arch the small of your back. Now, the first objective is to walk while holding this posture. Take a few steps (flats or stockinged feet please) and see how difficult it is.

Next, find a book of a reasonable size and weight. Balance the book on your head and walk forwards a few steps, turn, and walk back without dislodging it. If you look down, it will slip off. If you go too fast, it will jiggle off. If you lean too far back likewise. And if your stride is too long your balance won't be good and it will fall again. If you turn too fast your boob momentum or the sudden twist of your head sideways will dislodge the book again. Wear a skirt or dress with a tighter hemline to restrict your stride length. If you push against the material this will also baulk your progress which will, guess what, dislodge the book.

Practice till you can walk backwards and forwards and turn comfortably without losing the book and don't look too stiff or awkward. For a smoother turn pivot on the ball of one foot. As you gain confidence pick up the speed a little to an easy walking pace. Try it with different hemlines to see how they restrict your movement.

Don't look down at your boobs or feet. Keep your gaze straight ahead. If you look down that tilts your head forward. The mass of your head combines with the boobs to tilt your line of action out of the front of your body. That will make you walk quicker to compensate or lean back to counterbalance. As you walk notice that your hips rotate slightly as the leg swings through to the next step. This will make your boobs move from side to side. If you walk too quickly, they will start to get their own momentum. This is made worse if your stride is too long. When you run, they will jiggle up and down in reaction to your foot fall. We'll fix all that below.

Top tip: the whole exercise is easier if you keep your knees reasonably close together and take smaller steps. A knee length skirt tight on the leg will enforce this rule.

Standing (flamingo and T-bar)

Our next postural lesson is on standing. We look at standing for two reasons. First it is an opportunity to show off your curves and second if you are on your feet a lot you need a way to relieve the pressure from wearing heels.

A general rule is not to have your feet too wide, certainly less than a shoulder width apart. Standing wide footed with your hands on your hips is a power stance and more male. It will look particularly mannish if your skirt is not very wide and is stretched by your legs. We want something more receptive and modest, that means a more passive stance.

The flamingo is an easy pose and so called because it resembles a flamingo standing on one leg. Put your weight on one foot to create a supporting leg with the line of action through it for balance. Now bend your knee slightly on the other (non-weight bearing) leg. This will take the pressure off your foot. Don't lift the foot off the ground completely. Rest the heel by keeping the toe of the shoe in slight contact with the ground. Switch to the other leg when the supporting leg gets tired. Just like a flamingo. They also do it, by the way, to rest their legs.

You can get a classic female pose from this by noticing that the non-weight leg will sag forward and allow the hip to drop. The weight bearing hip will be higher. Raise the shoulder on the opposite side of the highest hip and twist your upper torso slightly toward the non-weight bearing side. This is a classic S-shaped three-quarter pose that you'll see in lots of fashion magazines. Slip a hand loosely onto your hip on one side or the other. This gives you some width but draws attention to your curves and waist. A more powerful pose is to put you hand on your waist.

The resting leg can move slightly out to the side, the front, or a little to the back in this pose but always keep it easily inside you skirt width and/or close to your weight bearing knee. If you keep the legs together with the resting leg knee slightly forward or across the other leg you get a particularly feminine look.

The T-bar: is our next position and a staple of show girls, pageant contestants, models, flight attendants and promotional advertising eye-candy all over the world. Again, it gives a flattering and pleasing shape to your body. It works by placing your feet in a T shape with one heel next to the arch of the other foot.

Choose one foot and turn it to face away from the forward position and out to the side at a slight angle (45 degrees max). This is the cross bar on the T. Put your weight on that foot and then bring the other foot in front of it so that it is at ninety degrees with the heel next to the arch. This makes the T shape. The line of action is through the cross point on the T so it a very relaxed and comfortable position.

Again, the weight bearing hip will be slightly higher compared to the other. Alter the tilt of the free hip by bending or relaxing the knee of the front foot. You'll also find that this twists your upper body. This little manoeuvre makes your bust look fuller and more pointed. It will certainly stretch any fabric across your chest. You may also notice that one shoulder is slightly raised compared to another. Slip a hand onto your hip and you have another classic pose.

Loose hands: when you pose don't let your hands just hang loose give them something to do. Hold the strap on your handbag or a pair of gloves. Put a hand loosely on your hip or waist (hip is more natural and girly). If you have a fuller dress hold the skirt material with one hand and swish or play with it coyly pulling it out to the side or just toy with it. Very cute and feminine that one.

In modelling there is also a thing called open hands. You will never see a model with a closed fist. Always keep the hands open with the fingers slightly apart unless you are showing off your manicure and jewellery. Another thing to try is to flick your wrist out in the pose so it gives the impression of airy movement. Alternatively hold your hands loosely in your lap. Have some fun with it.

Practice all these positions in the mirror until you can change stance between them smoothly and easily. Since our next topic is walking in heels you might as well put on a pair and get used to standing this way. That will build up your muscle and balance memory. Do it with a little flair and try tilting your head slightly to the side, down or looking off into the mid distance. This is how models pose in fashion magazines. Try different sized heels so that you can experience the nuances of balance and be more aware of your centre of gravity and line of action.

Walking in heels

Walking is a deliberate disturbance of our body balance which is controlled by alternating the line of action through opposite legs, so we don't fall over. This means we shift our weight bearing position in a two-stage process called the gait cycle. The first (or stance) phase last for 60% of the cycle and the second (or swing) phase lasts 40% of the time. See Figure 11. Let's look at both of these and then make modifications to allow for walking in heels.

Because we walk quickly and unconsciously most people think we just put our feet flat on the ground at each step and that is all. If you do that, you'll look very flat-footed. If you do it in heels, you'll look gawky and be unbalanced. Another misconception is that because you are more on the balls of your feet in heels you should put your toes down first. That's okay for running and pivoting movements but not for walking.

Let's get back to basics. In the first phase of the gait cycle the non-weight bearing leg swings forward. The heel makes contact with the ground first. Then the foot goes flat onto the ground. Then we start to transfer the weight into it and forward (this is called the midstance). Then we push off by lifting the heel to tip our weight forward and spring off the toes. In phase two we swing the opposite leg forward. We place the heel down and as it goes flat (midswing) the weight enters into the foot. This brings us back to our starting position but a little further forward.

Try this without your heels in slow motion so you can identify the parts of the cycle then speed it up. You may notice that your arms have a natural tendency to swing. We'll look at that in more detail in a moment. For now, get use to the rhythm. Once you are happy put on a pair of smaller heels (inch or two). Now try it again.

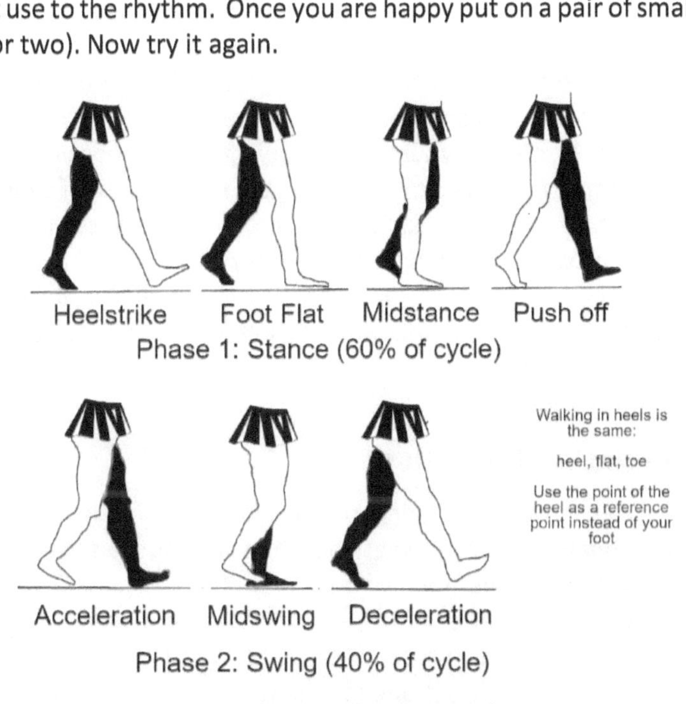

Figure 11 The two-phase gait cycle

In phase one, on the heel strike just touch the tip of the shoe heel lightly onto the ground. Use it to guide your foot flat. Take the weight on the leg (midstance) and then lift the heel to push off with your toes. Push off is the end of phase one. You may notice that the back of your other foot is already raised and ready to swing. In phase 2, accelerate the free foot through and past your other. Place the heel on the ground as a guide so that your foot can go flat and take the weight. Lift the heel to push-off and bring the original leg back off the ground ready for the next swing and heel strike. Do it quicker in phase 2 but not so much that it looks like you are uneven or limping.

Remember the height on the heels pushes your centre of gravity backwards. The tendency is to think that you have to arch the small of your back and lean back to stay upright and so the heel can clear the ground. It doesn't need to do this your feet are still at the same level just higher up. The natural bend and swing of your leg will give enough clearance. Keep that upright posture we practiced earlier: back straight and tummy tucked in. Look straight ahead (not down that will tip you forward) and intuitively feel when the heel touches the ground.

The difference between the usual gait and walking in heels is that you use the point of the heel as the guide not your foot. Don't put a lot of weight on the heel it is just a guide to ground you. You'll find this easier if you take smaller steps so the heel is more under your frame and you can rotate over it to place your foot. The weight comes as your foot goes flat and acts through the ball of your foot so you can push off again. The higher the heel the shorter your stride needs to be. Otherwise you won't be able to rotate properly. If you fight this and try to make big steps, you'll end up having to go straight to the flat stage and guess what you'll look gawky. Or worse the controlled accelerate and decelerate will get out of step and you'll catch the heel or fall over. Those little dainty steps are much more feminine anyhow and you'll feel more in control.

Hip sway and Rotation

Okay, now we are going to make your walk a little sexier. Women like to wear heels because it gives their hips and butt an extra little shimmy. This is just an exaggeration of a natural effect of pelvic rotation. Women have a wider and flatter pelvis, so it is more noticeable. Men do it as well because it is the most energy efficient way to walk. The difference in movement between male and female is only about 2 inches on either side, so it is well within your capacity.

Back to the biomechanics. When we walk, we swing our legs forwards effectively on two parallel tram lines about a shoulder width apart in our direction of travel. See Figure 12. The left and the right foot placement create a zig zag pattern between the two lines connecting our foot fall showing how we move forward. We get a longer stride and more energy efficient movement if we rotate the pelvis along with the leg swing. The rotation shifts our centre of gravity a little left and right so the hips sway to keep us balanced and the line of action through the weight bearing leg.

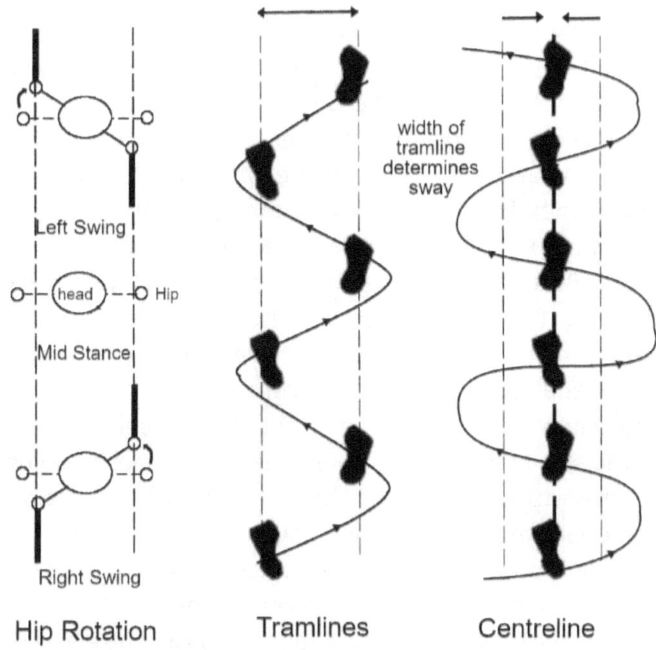

Figure 12 hip rotation and sway (using the centreline)

The body compensates for this with a few posture adjustments. You may notice that the upper body starts to rotate left and right as well. This is opposite to the twist of the pelvis. As the leg swings through you might also feel a slight rotation of the thigh bone and a twist of the ankle. Notice whether you put your foot down straight or whether it points off to the side. When you make the heel strike and then rotate into the flat position this can upset your balance. Instead of going straight over the heel to flat you rotate the ankle sideways so that the foot pivots around the heel onto the flat position. If the rotation doesn't complete, then you end up with your toes pointing slightly outwards. Duck feet.

To solve this misalignment and to exaggerate your sway we rotate the pelvis a little more than usual. All you need to do is bring those parallel tramlines closer together. This will allow your foot more time to rotate at the ankle so that your toes are pointing straight ahead. Much more femme. Let your hips go loose and don't resist the pelvic movement and you'll get some hip sway. The extreme of this position is for the left and right

147

tramlines to meet in the middle. In this case there is only a centre line and you aim to place both the left and right foot onto this centreline. This still keeps you well balanced but increases hip sway.

Try it now. Walk forward putting each foot on a centre line in front of you. Take it slow at first till you get used to the new balance position and then speed it up. Notice that the extra hip rotation means that you don't have to put so much effort into swinging the leg forward. Unchecked this will lengthen your stride. With those little dainty steps most of the movement comes from the hips and the leg swing is more about foot placement. Make sure your toes always point straight ahead when they are in midstance. Because your weight bearing leg is on the centre line you will have to swing the free leg around it. And that's even more sway. Experiment with different stride patterns until you get one that is comfortable, and you feel the most secure.

Notice how this varies as the height of your heel increases. Often you can keep the same stride pattern with the higher heel by doing more with your hips even though you need to be more careful placing your foot. Catwalk models exaggerate this movement even more. To get that fashionista look push your tramlines further so that they crossover the centre line. The right side is left of the centre and the left is right of centre. Practically this means that your foot falls just past centre and the swing leg crosses in front of the weight bearing leg. Not too much though because that looks wild and uncontrolled and you'll fall over yourself if you go too fast.

Practice this to get comfortable and combine it with the standing exercises. Imagine walking up the catwalk, pose (flamingo or T-bar), turn and walk back, pose and so on until you get the rhythm. With a bit of speed this will make your boobs sway with your upper body movement. Now you're all moving curves. Hey girl, you got a sexy shimmy going on!

Arm swing, Angulation and Bounce (the H-factor)

The next task is to control that side to side boob swing and then add some airiness to your walk. In the first case the movement is caused by the hip rotation and if it gets too exaggerated it will appear as though you are pointing your chest as you walk. Look at my boobies everyone. Arm swing is the way to control this but if it gets too rigid, you'll look like a fembot. We also want to give you a little bounce that will make you look light footed and delicate.

Arm swing: We swing our arms naturally when we walk to counteract all that angular momentum caused by hip sway. If you haven't noticed there is a particular pattern that synchronises with your leg movement. Imagine you had a bird's eye view of your walk looking directly down over your head. Your posture will look like the letter H. See Figure 13. The crossbar is your torso with the head in the middle and your hips at the edges. The two verticals are aligned to your normal tramlines when you walk. Your feet will always be at opposite corners of the H when you heel strike or push-off. And, for the best balance and least amount of boob swing your hands should be at the other corners.

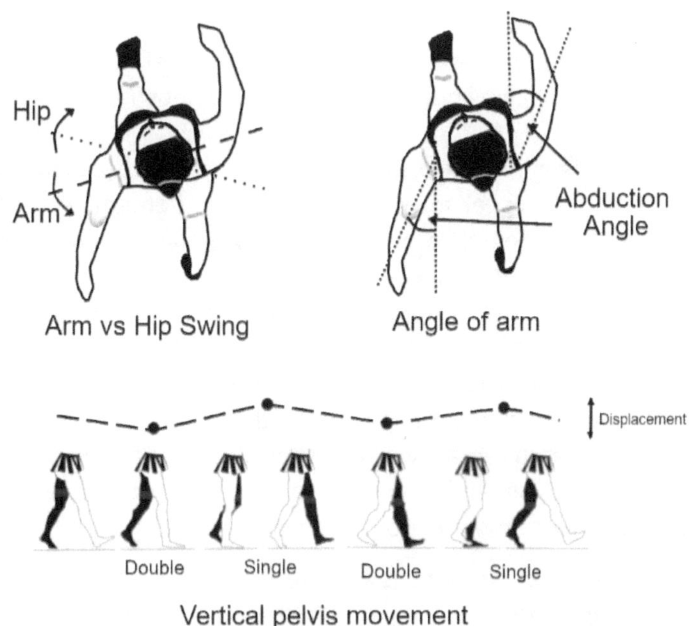

Figure 13 Arm swing and bounce

Walk it through slowly. Take a right step forward and let your left arm join it out front. The left foot will be behind you and let your right arm join it out back. See the H-shape. Now as you swing the left foot forward allow both arms to come back to your sides (this is mid-swing in phase 2 of the gait cycle). As the left foot goes out front with the right arm, the right foot moves to the back by virtue of the push off, so allow the left arm to join it. Now walk forwards keeping the rhythm. It's easier than it sounds.

The idea is that the rotation caused by the hip and leg in your lower half is matched by an opposite (counter) rotation of your shoulders and arm in the upper half of your body. So left leg matched by right arm and right leg matched by left arm. Get it. If you do it right, you'll be marching like a soldier. Your boobs will still move but much more gently and stay more or less pointing forward. The trick now is to relax that movement so that it looks more casual. Fortunately, girls have another trick up their sleeves.

Arm angulation: Have you ever wondered how those ice skaters manage to spin faster and faster on the spot? It is all to do with angular momentum and centrifugal forces. If you are spinning and stick your arms out, you'll slow down. If you pull your arms in your will speed up. Our hip rotation when we walk also works like this except that we don't spin all the way around and don't move as fast. We can be more effective in countering our boob swing by sticking our arms out a bit and not straight forward and back like a solider.

The angle your arm makes with your torso is called the abduction angle. And, it is bigger for women than men. Remember in chapter 2 we pointed out that female arms have more angulated elbows. This is so they can avoid the wider hips when they swing backwards and forwards. Their arm swing is not straight up and down on the tramlines of the H. Instead they flare out a little on the backward swing. This means you can be more relaxed and easier with your arm movement and it will still counteract the hip rotation. Let your arms go free and easy and flare a little as they go back. If you watch female walkers, they also have a freer wrist movement. Try your walk again and now let your arms swing girl style. Not too much. Just enough to stop the boob movement.

Bounce: the next element is to give your walk a little bounce. Catwalk models exaggerate this quite a bit and you see their hips dipping as well as swaying when they walk. It can look almost like a flounce. The trick to this movement is simple when you understand the biomechanics.

As we walk our pelvis doesn't just rotate it also moves up and down. It allows us to compensate for undulations in the surface we are walking on. We tend to miss this part of our gait because we now more or less always walk on flat floors. The pelvis is highest when we are bearing all the weight on a single leg and lowest when we support the weight with both legs. It is at its highest when we are in midstance and transferring the weight into the foot (see Figure 13). You can get a better feel for this with a wider stride. The greater the step the more your pelvis will drop as the legs flex to transfer the weight from single to double support and back again. Try it (without your heels) and you'll look like someone from the ministry of silly walks.

Because we are using smaller steps in our heels this up and down movement is reduced but you can bring it back by flexing your knee. By the way you should never lock your knees when you are walking in heels always have a bit of flex in them. When you walk give an extra little push on the push-off by flexing your knee. On the heel strike relax your knee a little more allowing the leg (and hip) to sink more onto the foot. Takes a little practice this one but when you coordinate the two your hips will bounce a little more and your walk will have an airier feel. If you are wearing a lighter fuller (knee length) skirt this action will cause a little sympathetic motion in the material which looks lovely and feminine.

Okay so now let's put it all together. Start your walk and then swing the arms with that little outward flare and as you pick up some momentum start flexing your knees. Back it off a little until it looks natural and you have a nice feminine walk with hip sway, bounce, and some hand movement. Notice that your boobs also have a little movement but not too much. Lovely. Exaggerate the individual components and you can be that sultry catwalk model. Enjoy!

Stairs, Slopes and other things

We have learned all we can from the biomechanics and constructed a female walk. What next? Well that kind of walk only works effectively on a fairly even surface. You'll need a few more skills if you are to navigate effectively down the street, in the office block, or have fun in your heels.

Stairs: walking up and down stairs can seem like a daunting task because the heels elevate you forward onto your toes and balance you on a point. When you look over the edge of a stairwell you might take a gulp. Fortunately, it is easier than it looks. Turn a little sideways and put your whole foot down flat onto the next step down. Use the heel a little for a guide on the drop if you need to and then put your foot down. Don't rotate just go flat. The surface is lower than you are so it should be easy.

You turn sideways a little so that you can get both the heel and ball down evenly at the same time. If you are concentrating on getting the heel down it will be ahead of the rest of your foot which is not good and you can miss place the front of your foot on the edge of the tread so that you will slip off when you transfer the weight. This is especially true if the stairs treads are narrow. If there is a stair rail use it to steady yourself, just in case. Much better than missing a step, tripping, and shooting down the stairs. If you do get into trouble steady yourself with the rail or sit on the step to recover. This is much more dignified than skirts flying.

Going upstairs is much easier. Just put the ball and toe of your foot onto the front of the step and leave the heel free. Use your push-off to gain the height for the next step. Hold the railing and you can help with this. And, flex your knee a little to add some bounce. It's like a little run upstairs on tiptoes.

Slopes: any surface with an incline is a nightmare for heels. Take the stairs next to a ramp or find another route. If the incline is very tiny (barely noticeable) you should be okay but even a modest slope can cause problems. You might be forced to run down one to keep your balance and bend over ungainly to get up one.

The issue is that your heels tilt your foot which affects your tipping point. Imagine a tall, thin rectangular box and try to push it over. One of the side edges will become a pivot point. As you push, the box will reach a critical angle and then will fall over under its own weight. This crucial angle depends on two things. The centre of gravity and the width of the box. The higher the centre of gravity the smaller the angle of the tipping point. If you pack a box and put all the light things at the bottom it will be easier to tip over than if you put all the heavy things at the bottom. Guess what, our bodies are packed with the heavy things at the top.

What has all this got to do with heels and slopes. Well, you're like a thin tall box with a narrow width and the cog at the top. Your heels make your centre of gravity higher and tip you onto your toes. The line of action is close to the front of the box. The tipping angle depends on the length of your foot and the height of the heel. The height is the difference between the underside of the ball of your foot and the underside of the heel. These horizontal and vertical measurements form a right-angled triangle. Typical high heels give your foot an angle of 20-40 degrees.

Now can you see the problem with slopes? If your tipping point was 45 degrees (and it's probably less). Then a 5-degree slope is more than you can manage in the highest heel. You will fall over no matter how careful you are. For the smallest heels you can only cope with a 25-degree slope since the 20 degrees from your heels gets added to the angle of the slope (that is, 20+25).

To put that into terms you can visualise a 45-degree slope is a 1-1 ratio so there is a one foot change in height for every foot forward. A 25-degree slope is more like one foot change for four feet forward. And a 5-degree slope is one foot for every twenty feet. So even small inclines need your attention when your heels are high.

Going downhill you might try to compensate by leaning back. That might be okay for a small incline and low heels but since you are just a thin box (in our analogy) you are just as likely to fall backwards. A better strategy is to accept you are unbalanced and try to run down. If its short and not too steep you might get away with this. Going uphill you might think you can lean forward a little. Yes, you can but it is ungainly and above a certain gradient your heels will slip and you will fall forward probably skinning your knees. Alternatively, you might try to tack up or down the slope sideways like a skier on a snowy mountain. Very ungainly. All in all, it is just too much hassle so avoid slopes.

Unfortunately, men friends, in their flat shoes don't think like this. On a night out you might be left stranded. Time to play your girl card and ask for some gallant help. If you cannot do that use the railing if there is one or take your heels off. Imagine that romantic walk on the beach, heels in one hand, holding hands with the other and feeling the sand on your bare feet.

Running and Dancing

Our last topic in this section is running and dancing. These might seem like strange bedfellows, but they require the same technique. That is, stay on the balls of your feet and avoid contact of the heel points with the ground.

If you need to hurry along keep your feet (toes) on the centre line and let your foot swing out to the side and back under you. This will avoid your unconscious expectation to put your heel down first like walking. If you do the latter it will twist your ankle, break the heel, or do both. If your skirt is narrow you won't be able to extend into a full stride, so the side swing is a little dainty movement to quicken the pace. Notice if you go too fast your boobs will move up and down excessively.

Likewise, if you are dancing and put too much weight on the heel by lifting the front of your foot. That will tip you over backwards or break the heel. You need lighter feet. When you dance put the heel back just to ground yourself if you need to but always aim to keep the majority through the front of your foot. This allows you to pivot and spin but also to step back. If you can dance the Charleston in your heels you have mastered this technique.

Try this at home until you are super confident. Do your walk. As you come to a stop take a step back into a T-bar position. Hand on hip and pose. Then pivot on the ball of one foot and walk in the opposite direction and repeat. If you have enough room walk a triangle. Once you have this down put on some music and dance to the tune. If you have any difficulties reduce the heel height or get a shoe with more support. If you can, dance with a partner, hold hands and practise moving backwards and forwards to the tune and doing a twirl.

Sitting Properly

Women have several ways to sit and arrange their legs. All these techniques are designed to keep your knees together and preserve your modesty. Pantie flashing has become a bit of a controversial subject of late with the suggestion that some women do it deliberately as an attraction signal. Think Sharon Stone in that notorious scene from *Basic Instinct*. Mostly though it is an action of the ingenue. For example, Selma Blair as Cecile Caldwell in the cult movie, *Cruel intentions*. Adopt the following techniques and you'll always retain your dignity.

Leg arrangement: Depending on the height and softness of what you are sitting on your bottom will sink into the fabric and your knees will come up higher than your hips. This is worse when you are wearing heels because the heel adds height to your knee. Your skirt hem and the gap between your knees will tilt upwards at the correct angle for anyone curious to take a look. Modesty says you should avoid this. With the chance of people seeing your tuck or lack of one you'll have extra incentive.

The easiest way to avoid embarrassment is to keep your knees together. You can do this by having the whole of your inner legs pressed slightly together or just the tops to your knees with your lower legs at an angle. The latter looks a little cute especially if you turn in your ankles.

A way to bring your knees level with your hips and avoid awkwardness is to tilt your legs sideways. With your inner legs touching and knees together, this makes a classic female look. It is also practical because you can balance a handbag, gloves, papers, laptop, or drink on your upper legs. A variation is to hook one foot behind the other at the ankle. This works very well in heels. If you are waiting for someone it is also a chance to show off your manicure and nails. Place your hands palm down with one slightly overlapping the other in your lap. One hand on each leg is more like man hands.

The foot dangle: An alternative leg posture is to cross one leg over the other at the knee. This closes off the upskirt problem but also allows your foot to dangle. This will show off your stockings, heels and your nicely shaped calf. With some ankle decoration or seam this can look very classy. If your shoes are looser you can also slip the heel letting the shoe dangle casually from your toes which is seen as quite relaxed and highly sensual. There is something about the bare foot in stockings. For a more pleasing and comfortable line tilt the leg of the non-dangling foot so your heel is not flat on the floor.

Getting up and down: the next challenge is getting up from or down to a sitting position with grace and elegance. Stand at a slight angle to the seat and place one foot slightly in front of the other. As you start to sit, twist the pelvis in to bring your knees together and then down to place your tush on the seat. With relatively little practice this can be done in a nice fluid movement. You will find that the legs fall almost naturally into one for those demure arrangements we just discussed.

However, there is one additional thing to remember. As you drop down into the seat trace a hand along the curve of your bottom to the top of the legs to smooth the skirt material flat before you sit. This is a little nicety that works for fuller skirts and for petticoats. It stops them ruching and leaving unsightly skirt folds or ballooning up for that upskirt effect. It also ensures that when you stand the material won't have creased or not fall correctly back around your legs. It doesn't matter so much for tighter skirts but is still a nice feminine gesture.

Once you are down on the seat either stay perched with an upright posture on the front or slide back to a more comfortable position. Don't perch and let the shoulders slump. And don't slouch if you push back. That just offers the cleavage or shots of your bra or forms to anyone passing by.

Boy Bending versus Girl Bending

Our last piece of advice can be summarized by the pithy phrase: dirty girls bend at the waist; good girls bend at the knees. Bending at the waist is something you are used to as a male but girls use their knees. One reason for this is that bending at the waist is a sure way to flash your panties in a short skirt or display your bust by tipping it forward. Bending at the waist like this is a staple of glamour model posing usually accompanied with a cheeky or suggestive look over the shoulder. These are okay for playboy or the bedroom but not when you are out and about.

It is not just about modesty though. A study in the journal *Gait and Posture* by Valentina Graci and colleagues, from University of Maryland, Washington University, and St. Louis University showed that there were specific differences in the way men and women perform a one-legged squat. Bending at the knees is similar but not identical to a one-legged squat but we can still learn something from the study.

Women hold their upper body more upright than men who tend to lean forward. Both have to keep the centre of mass over the supporting foot to stay in balance, but they do it differently. In a female squat the shoulders and hip remain aligned vertically forming a pillar of strength. Men bend more at the waist, and push the buttocks out, forming a triangle between shoulder, hip, and foot. Obviously sticking your butt out like this is more pin-up style.

These differences require other changes too. Women flex their trunks toward the weight bearing leg as they lower straight down over the foot. Men do the opposite, flexing the upper body to the non-weight bearing leg. Both methods keep the upper body balanced and the line of action through the supporting leg. Men move their trunk to use upper and lower body as counterweights. Women don't need to do this. The main difference is that females rotate the pelvis towards the weight bearing leg while males rotate the opposite way. As a result, men demand more from their hip muscles whereas women demand more of their knee muscles. From a modesty point of view, one closes and the other opens your legs.

Try it and see which way you twist your pelvis and upper body. Are you doing the male or female version? Ideally, keep your legs close together with one foot slightly further forward than the other. Take more weight on your front leg and as you squat, twist the pelvis towards the forward leg so that the knees come together. The back leg might go onto tip toes as you twist with the heel supporting your bottom. That's okay it makes it easier when you are wearing heels. Retrieve your item (or whatever) and then reverse. Push up off the knees, balance weight in both legs (bring the heel of the back leg down) and then push up from the knees.

The beauty of this technique is that it works for tight as well as loose skirts or dresses. As you twist inwards you keep your knees together so that closes off any inadvertent upskirt view from the front even for quite short skirts. Likewise, by resting on your opposite heel you take pressure off your knees and cover a back upskirt view. If you twist the opposite way (like a man) you will open your legs and flash your panties.

Since your trunk is upright throughout you also minimise the chance of inadvertently displaying more of your cleavage than intended. If you can, perform the whole operation quickly so you are not down there for too long. A quick bob down and up looks like a kind of curtsey.

Top tip: you might find you have bias to one side or the other which makes bending easier.

Practise List

There is no shopping list for this chapter instead we have a practice list. You can integrate all these exercises with your normal activities around the house. This will also wear your heels in so they are more comfortable for longer periods and the sole is roughed a little and not slippy.

Maintain an upright posture
Always bend at the knees not the waist
Always sit with your legs together (whole legs together or tops to knees with lower legs apart)
Practice crossing your legs in a variety of ways (tilt your legs sideways and adjust your hem)
Practice perching (sit on the chair arm or against a desk or table)
Rest your feet with the flamingo and T-bar (when doing chores or when you are on the phone)
Pose in front of the mirror (imagine you are on a photoshoot and go through your poses)
Practice turning and transitioning from stand to walk, sitting and bending
Practice your catwalk sway and bounce
Practice walking on different surfaces (carpet, tiles, lino, polished wood, tarmac)
Practice going up and down stairs
And, of course, dance to your favourite tunes.

To avoid mishap only wear a heel as high as you feel comfortable in. If you cannot manage the heel at home don't wear it out. A shoe that covers your foot and gives extra support and a wider heel point is better at first till you get all your manoeuvres down. As you go up in height look for a strappy kind of shoe this will balance joint flexibility with more support so that you minimise slip and movement of the shoe on the foot which can cause you to misstep.

When you take each step, or if you feel yourself slipping, arch your foot slightly to put pressure on the inside of your shoe. This will make your shoe fit closer and make it easier to control your movements. If you do get the wobbles stop and gather yourself. Don't press on or you run the risk of turning an ankle. Connect back with your centre of gravity and then step out again. Make such pauses look more natural by adjusting your skirt or dress, smoothing down the line, checking your stocking seams or your handbag before continuing.

When walking outdoors be extra vigilant for the type of surface. Avoid uneven surfaces if you can or places where there are grilles or cracks in pavement slabs. Dips and cracks are a magnet for narrow heel points and even a slight unevenness will give you a balance problem. If you do need to venture across a problem area do it slow and pick your way through. Otherwise you'll stumble or get your heel stuck or even break it off. If the latter happens, you'll twist or sprain your ankle if you're lucky and be in casualty on crutches if you're not. All the above is extra pertinent when you have to hurry for something like a taxi and forget yourself. Drainage grilles or manhole covers at the edge of the roadside are so easy to miss and they are a real heel trap.

Indoors watch for the transition from carpet to tiles or polished wood. These surfaces have different levels of friction and the bottom of heeled shoes by and large don't have much grip or tread. If the surface has less grip smaller steps are required so that you can get heel to flat to push off without slipping. On carpets the depth of pile will allow the heel point to sink so you must lift and push off properly to avoid snagging the surface. If the carpet is deep, it's an uneven surface (see above) try and walk around it or take your heels off. A smaller step will keep your line of action closer to your torso. If someone offers you a supportive hand be ladylike and accept. Hold their forearm or hand. Don't loll all over them.

And finally …

That all seems like a lot to remember except that it isn't. If you practice regularly and maintain the right posture you will develop muscle memory, and everything will become unconscious. Practice really is the key. Don't go mad at it though just walking and bending in heels can be fatiguing until you build up the muscles. Two hours around the house in heels will leave your calves and leg muscles aching. The higher the heel and the narrower the tip the more pressure they put on your legs and toes.

Make sure you pamper yourself with a muscle soak and let your legs recover.

That's another way of saying don't rush into your highest heels. Yes, we know. You want the biggest heels and the shortest dress for clubbing! Work up with smaller heels to get your confidence. A platform shoe might not be as sexy but it will give you the height to practice with more support for your foot. And, in the long run you'll be much more comfortable on your pins.

If you can walk okay in lower heels but find that in the higher ones you still have problems, it might not just be a question of balance. Some shoes will just be too high for you. Remember that critical angle? The tipping point depends on the angle made by the ratio of your foot length and the difference in height between the ball and heel of your foot. It is greater if your feet are smaller. Beyond a certain ratio you will be close to your tipping point (40+ degrees) which will make any movements, sways, or nudges push you off balance. You can get the same height without the uncertainty by using a platform shoe. The extra thickness of the platform is deducted from your ball to heel height and reduces your critical angle. Platforms give you height with more stability.

When you wear heels the back of your ankle and calf elongate giving you a longer slimmer look. A lot of women want that elegant profile but you have to learn to compensate for the extra pressure on your feet. If you habitually wear heels (especially high ones) the calf muscles shorten while the ankle muscles stretch to compensate. Eventually you will find it difficult to walk normally and won't be able to wear flat shoes at all. The steeper the angle of the foot the more pressure is placed on the toes. Like a ballet dancer doing pointe if this is a regular position you will damage, break or distort your toes. Watch or train your posture as we suggest above and take regular time out in flats or lower heels to keep the muscles in the right proportions.

And last, practice till you get a nice feminine flow to your walk that will allow you to fit into your surroundings. We have mentioned lots of ways to adjust your movement and walk from bounce to hip sway and how to deport yourself. The number one give away for crossdressers and Tgirls is to overdo your walk for the situation. Either it is too airy or flouncy or there is too much hip rotation or sway, or you look like a catwalk model wherever you go. Remember that models exaggerate everything. This is fine for a photoshoot or a fashion show but not when you are out and about. The word for this is mincing or to be affectively dainty or effeminate. Unless you are roleplaying don't mince, okay.

Chapter 10 Summary

Well, that's it, darlings! Everything you need to know to get your femme body in shape. Whether you are new to crossdressing or have some experience, I hope that you have found a little something to take away. Even if that is only a bit more appreciation for the wonders of the female form.

In the first part of the book we encouraged you to think about your motivations for dressing whether that is for fun, for social reasons, or part of something more permanent. A large part of enjoying your dressing is to get in touch with your feminine side and to find out what the inner you needs to feel happy and loved. Hopefully as you have mulled over the topics in this book you have learned to listen to that inner voice and have a much better idea of the things she likes and the look you want.

We encouraged you to think about the idea of a makeover to try out new things and to immerse yourself in a day to indulge your inner longings and wear clothes that it might not be economic for you to buy yourself. The advantage of that approach is that you can work with a sympathetic person to try out your look and to get the full ensemble of body, clothes, hair and makeup just right. This will give you a window into the future, an advanced snapshot, if you will, of the way you could be when you have perfected all your dressing techniques.

We also gave you a pamper routine to help feminize your body but also to indulge your inner girl. Even if your dressing is an occasional activity paying attention to all the little things like hair removal, moisturising, and keeping your nails neat and trimmed will allow you to enjoy being feminine. There is nothing like the feel of silky soft skin and nice under things or for that matter looser women's attire when you are alone for the evening. If you want to you can limit your dressing just to underwear under your normal clothes or male lingerie. Whatever floats your boat.

In part 2 attention shifted onto body types and what you can do to have a more pleasing feminine shape. We learned the importance of keeping your curves in proportion and looked at ways to enhance your form. We also considered ways to give you a perfect pair of boobs using a variety of techniques. How to enhance your butt so it looks nice and round, as well as hiding your male bits to give that perfect Y shape at the front. How much you want or need to apply these techniques depends on what you want to achieve with your dressing and the kind of clothes you want to wear. We gave you some shopping lists but also some DIY tips for those managing on a budget.

Part 3 moved the focus on to the types of clothes and materials available to your feminine persona and how these could be used to enhance your look or hide difficult features. We looked at the essentials of your intimate attire and how fashion and fads help or hinder looking feminine. The right cuts of clothing, patterning, and embellishments are all important and help to define your individuality and look. Last but definitely not least, we looked at deportment and movement. How your centre of gravity is changed when you add boobs to your chest or add height to your feet with heels. We looked at ways to sit, stand, and bend. In considering the biomechanics of walking we retrained your body so that you could walk and move elegantly in heels. The idea of a demure gait and posture is something that is quintessentially feminine. You learned all the secrets and now need practice. Develop the muscle memory and instinctiveness that makes such movements unconscious.

And finally, you may be a little disappointed that we didn't touch on that important topic of makeup and hair styling. This has been primarily a body book. Yes, your head and face are part of your body but they require such attention that they can only be treated adequately with a separate volume. Neither did we talk about that important aspect of your female persona, your voice. If you enjoyed this book, I hope you will look out for the sister volumes that cover these last two topics in more detail.

Au revoir for now and do enjoy your dressing in whatever form it takes.

Resources

There are a huge variety of clothing retailers online and in the high street. Below are some places, ideas and options to build your wardrobe that may not be that easy to find. Note that not all these places are crossdressing aware. Act in a discreet manner when dealing with any staff or help desks.

Popular sites such as ebay, etsy, amazon, and ASOS also carry a huge range of affordable clothing, styles, and accessories for crossdressing if you know what you are looking for as well as mainstream female clothing for all ages.

Crossdressing supplies

Range of crossdressing clothing and padding: https://enfemmestyle.com
Range of Body shaping and Breastforms: https://www.glamourboutique.com
Range of shoes, stockings, and lingerie: https://crossdressingcloset.com
Wide range of clothing designed for crossdressers: https://janetscloset.com
Just about everything including leather & PVC: www.crossdressboutique.com

Plus size

D-K cup clothing https://www.curvykate.com
Clothing and lingerie for curvy girls: https://www.simplybe.co.uk
Plus-size intimates: https://www.hipsandcurves.com
Size 16-28 clothes https://pinkclove.co.uk
Plus Size and shapewear https://naturalcurves.co.uk

Retro Look

1900-1960 Vintage Fashion and beauty archive: https://glamourdaze.com
1900-1970s more vintage fashion: https://vintagedancer.com
1920s-1990s Fashion styles, Trends, pictures and history:
https://www.retrowaste.com
1800 -1900 Regency, Victorian, and Edwardian: https://www.fashion-era.com
Range of vintage dresses and petticoats: https://www.lindybop.co.uk
More Vintage dresses: https://www.ladyvlondon.com
Nice range of old style babydoll nighties https://myretrocloset.com

Fully fashioned stockings & Girdles

Genuine stockings in 1950s style: https://www.stockingshq.com
Range of Corsets, Girdles, and stockings https://www.truecorset.co.uk
Manufacturers of vintage lingerie (great range): https://www.nylon-dreams.co.uk
Huge collection stockings, tights, holdups and brand names:
https://www.mayfairstockings.com

Directoire Style

Knickers, corsetry, and slips: https://www.annettes-knickers.co.uk
Lingerie and Nightwear: https://www.slenderella.co.uk
Satin and lace sets and fuller panties: https://www.missdiscreet.com
Range of items: https://www.lingeriediva.com

Petticoats

Wide range of different types and some plus sizes: https://www.jjshouse.co.uk
Wide range uk size 6-26, swing & wiggle dresses:
https://www.dollyanddotty.co.uk
Beautiful handmade petticoats: https://www.dreampetticoats.co.uk
50s style and clothes: https://hellbunny.com

Sissy clothing

Maids & Sissy, Lingerie, Uniforms, mistress wear and more:
https://thedominatrixstore.com
Wide range of sissy clothes www.lingeriebychristine.co.uk
Lolita fashion clothing: https://www.lolitain.com

Men's lingerie

Men's lingerie: https://xdress.co.uk
Panties, Bras, and tops: https://shop.hommemystere.com
Huge range of tights from sheer to opaque: https://www.tights-for-men.com

Note: All URLs were live as of January 2020. As always take care shopping
or providing information online. Inclusion in the list does not indicate any
endorsement by the author.

Other Books By Martine

How To Feminize Your Voice, 2019, pp126

ISBN10: 1794084177, ISBN13:9781794084179,
ASIN: B07M85MTPY

Voice feminization is a growing phenomenon. This straightforward how-to-book provides all the tricks, tips, and advice you'll need to create a passable feminine voice. We start by creating your baseline femme voice and then build on it with resonance, rhythm and word choices to give you a voice that matches your personality. Each chapter provides a little theory, exercises, as well as things to avoid. Whether you want a temporary or permanent adjustment or are just curious to find out how female speakers use their voice differently to men there will be something of interest inside.

Martine's book is ideal for self-help. You can go at your own pace or work with friends. The book covers the techniques used by voice therapists and voice coaches to give your voice flexibility and to change how you pronounce words and to give you that characteristic female lilt. There are a few extra insights and visualizations to help things go more smoothly based on the authors experience. If a voice therapist is too expensive and the idea of throat surgery scares you this is a great way to get started on your femme voice.